ADVANCE PRAISE

Finally, a little handbook for all quality management professionals that addresses a very important subsystem in the quality management system—CAPA.
—*Helen Hughes, MBA, Manager CAPA Compliance*

Finally, a handbook with information that a person working on the shop floor can use! This book takes the big mystery out of CAPA! David Muchemu has done quality engineers, quality managers, and process engineers great service—information at your fingertips!
—*Dr Anthony Hall, Ph.D, Quality Systems Engineering Manager*

David Muchemu takes the fear and complications out of CAPA, something that is past due! This is a handbook every quality professional should have on his or her desk!
—*Tim Atkinson, CQE, MBA*

Profitability through compliance! What an idea! This book offers an understanding of CAPA from QSR and ISO quality system point of view. CAPA is the circulatory subsystem of any quality management system—what an idea!
—*Ayub Monte, MBA, Quality Systems Manager*

HOW TO DESIGN A WORLD-CLASS
Corrective Action Preventive Action
SYSTEM FOR FDA-REGULATED INDUSTRIES

A HANDBOOK FOR QUALITY ENGINEERS
AND QUALITY MANAGERS

by

DAVID N. MUCHEMU

Bloomington, IN 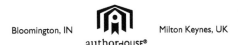 Milton Keynes, UK

authorHOUSE®

AuthorHouse™
1663 Liberty Drive, Suite 200
Bloomington, IN 47403
www.authorhouse.com
Phone: 1-800-839-8640

AuthorHouse™ UK Ltd.
500 Avebury Boulevard
Central Milton Keynes, MK9 2BE
www.authorhouse.co.uk
Phone: 08001974150

First published by AuthorHouse 8/16/2006

ISBN: 1-4259-5053-1 (sc)

Printed in the United States of America
Bloomington, Indiana

This book is printed on acid-free paper.

DEDICATION

This book is dedicated to the memory of Mister James Felix Wamoya, a brother and a friend who taught me the power of the rosary, the rewards of hard work, and the importance of family. May the Lord have mercy on your soul, grant you eternal life, and rest you in peace.

Also
To my mother, Mrs. Rachael Muchemu, for her tough love, her guidance through tough times, and her free counsel. I miss you, Mother.

And
To Peter Senge, who opened my eyes to systems approach to quality management, the effects of interactive loops within a quality management system, and the power and effects of system dynamics.

Finally
To the memory of Dr Edward Deming and to all the professionals in the pharmaceutical, medical device, biomedical, and cellular therapy industries who work hard to make quality products and provide quality services that improve the quality of the human condition around the globe. Yours is a worthy cause.

CONTENTS

■PREFACE

This book is written for three reasons: First, to take the myth out of CAPA. Second, to help quality professionals responsible for controlling the cost of quality through continuous process improvement design a CAPA quality subsystem that addresses both the reactive and proactive loops within any quality management system, with the emphasis being placed on the proactive loop. The purpose of the proactive loop is to improve the organization's profitability by catching mistakes before they happen. In the words of one FDA inspector, "Prevention is better than cure!" The proactive loop described in this book addresses that. For that reason, I have purposely put more emphasis on the proactive loop. In the more than the twenty years I have worked in cGMP environments, I have found that most organizations spend their resources putting out fires (reactive mode) rather than using those resources to actively look out for conditions that may set a fire ablaze (proactive mode). The information provided in this book should be used as a guide to the design of a robust CAPA system that meets both regulatory and business requirements, regardless of the product or service your organization provides. My third reason for writing this book is to help reduce the confusion surrounding CAPA. CAPA is a very simple quality subsystem that has been built into a monster shrouded in confusion and fear. To achieve that, I have used diagrams where necessary. It is my hope that I have achieved these three objectives.

David N.Muchemu, MBA.
President, Quality Systems International (QSI), a quality system and process improvement company
E-mail: muchemudaudi@yahoo.com
Office: (408) 429-3998

CHAPTER 1:
CAPA DEFINED

A CAPA system is ***not*** a database for problems, nor is it software for tracking problems and events that affect the quality management system (QMS). A CAPA system is a continuous process, product, and QMS improvement quality subsystem. Simply put, the mission of a CAPA subsystem is to continuously improve the products, process, and quality management system of any given organization, regardless of the product the organization specializes in. It accomplishes this mission through two quality loops: the "preventive loop" and the "corrective loop." The preventive action loop is proactive: It deals with adverse trends in the quality management system which, if left unattended, may lead to future problems. The second quality loop is the reactive loop. This loop deals with actual adverse events and problems that affect the product, process, and quality management system. The mission of this loop is to put out fires. It deals with actual problems that occur in the organization due to failures in trend detection in the preventive loop. In a layman's language: whereas the preventive loop deals with symptoms of a future decease, the corrective loop deals with the decease itself. Once identified, potential problems, events, and actual problems have to be prioritized for resource allocation. Different organizations have different ways of prioritizing problems.

Here is a summary of what a robust CAPA system achieves for an organization:

(a) It identifies all discrepancies, deviations, and non-conformance associated with the quality system, products, processes, and customer complaints.

(b) It identifies adverse trends related to process, product, quality system, and customers using statistical methods and risk analysis.

(c) It prioritizes quality problems for investigation based on the significance and the risk posed by the problem to the organization.

(d) It allows for traceability of non-conforming products, discrepancies, deviations, customer complaints, and other non-conformance.

(e) It allows for investigation of quality system problems, process problems, product problems, and customer complaints.

(f) It allows for investigations of adverse trends related to processes, products, and the quality system.

(g) It addresses both reactively and proactively problems related to processes, product, customers and the entire quality management system.

1

(h) It resolves all quality issues affecting the organization with levels of accountability and traceability.

(i) It incorporates new ways of doing things into the quality management system, and quality control with traceability, through a change control system.

The nine items mentioned above are business baseline requirements for any corrective action/preventive action system. The CAPA system serves as a continuous improvement heart of the quality management system. It is no accident that CAPA is the initial focus of all FDA audits. A good CAPA system tells the health of the quality system. As mentioned earlier, a CAPA system operates on two system loops: a reactive loop and a proactive loop. The two loops counter the effects of each other. In a more efficient system, there should be fewer CARs (Corrective Action Requests) coming into the system than PARs (Preventive Action Requests). The logic here is simple: "Prevention is better than cure." Potential problems should be addressed in the preventive loop before they become actual problems in the reactive loop. Potential problems show up in the form of trends and other risk analysis data like PFMEA or DFMEA. Trends and risk analysis data lead to the generation of Preventive Action Requests (PARs). Needless to say, this is the most important loop in your CAPA system. The corrective (reactive) loop only kicks in when the organization fails to identify potential problems in the preventive (proactive) loop. Problems and potential problems discovered in a CAPA system (discovery phase) are contained, investigated, and resolved in the reactive loop. Problems trigger a reaction in the system. The QMS (quality management system) merely reacts to the problem through an initiation of a CAR (Corrective Action Request). On the other hand, adverse trends or risk analysis data triggers the preventive loop of the CAPA system for system adjustment through a PAR (Preventive Action Request). This stops problems that may otherwise show up in the corrective action loop as crisis events, customer returns, process rejects, or recalls. The difference between corrective action and preventive action must be made clear. Here, preventive action is based on trends (statistical or otherwise). It is proactive. It aims at stopping *occurrence* of problems looming on the horizon—problems waiting to happen. Corrective, action on the other hand, is reactive and addresses actual problems at hand. Corrective action aims at stopping *reccurence* of problems that have already occurred.

A word of caution needs to be said here: There are other actions taken by organizations on a daily basis that affect their missions. These include

- Issue of Engineering Change Requests (ECRs), called Engineering Change Notes (ECNs) in some organizations

- Variance requests

- Planned deviation requests

These three should be monitored through the CAPA quality subsystem.

Essentially, any action that affects or has the potential to affect your processes, your quality management system, or your products should be monitored through your CAPA subsystem.

ANALOGY:

Like the human body, any quality management system comprises several subsystems. The ISO 9001 QMS has twenty quality subsystems, commonly referred to as articles. They are as follows:

4.1 Management responsibility
4.2 Quality system
4.3 Contract review
4.4 Design control
4.5 Document control
4.6 Purchasing
4.7 Control of customer-supplied products
4.9 Process control
4.10 Inspection and testing
4.11 Control of inspection, measuring, and testing equipment
4.12 Inspection and test status
4.13 Control of non-conforming products
4.14 Corrective and preventive action
4.15 Handling, storage, packaging, preservation, and delivery
4.16 Control of quality records
4.17 Internal quality audits
4.18 Training
4.19 Servicing
4.20 Statistical techniques

All these quality management subsystems, or articles as they are commonly referred to, work collectively to achieve the mission of the organization, which is meeting the requirements of external customers while maintaining profitability.

The human body (a system), on the other hand, comprises the following subsystems:

1. The respiratory system
2. The circulatory system
3. The nervous system
4. The reproductive system
5. The digestive system

At any given time, these five subsytems work collectively as a unit to achieve the desired human condition: health and procreation. The nervous system (management review system) continuously reviews data from other systems for adjustment. In most cGMP organizations, the management review subsystem receives external and internal data about the organization from the CAPA. The ISO9001 and 820 QSR quality management systems are not different. They both require all the subsystems, or articles, to function collectively as a unit to achieve customer satisfaction. The CAPA subsystem collects data on all subsystems, allows for immediate action when needed, or investigates. Specified owners accomplish all actions taken.

SYSTEM REPRESENTATION OF A CAPA SYSTEM:

A CAPA system operates on two counter loops:

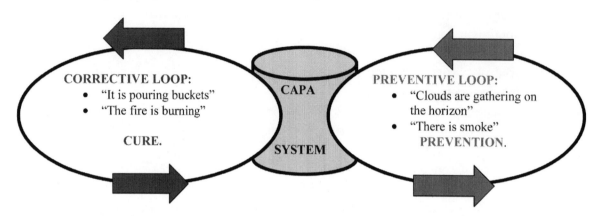

EXAMPLES:

- Low process yields
- High reject rates
- High cost of quality
- High scrap rate
- Customer complaints
- Process failures

EXAMPLES:

1. Drifting processes
2. Low process CPK
3. Fluctuating quality indicators

4. High PRN from DFM EA

There are two loops in operation at any given time. What you see in the corrective loop is the failure of what should have been caught in the preventive loop. In other words, if you are spending a lot of your time putting out fires, you are not investing resources in ***actively*** looking for potential problems in the preventive loop and stopping them from ***occurrence***.

■ CHAPTER 2:
CONCEPTUAL DESIGN

Methodically, draft a CAPA concept that paints a ***clear*** picture of what the system does and what it accomplishes.

A. THE CONCEPT: CONTINOUS IMPROVEMENT LOOPS

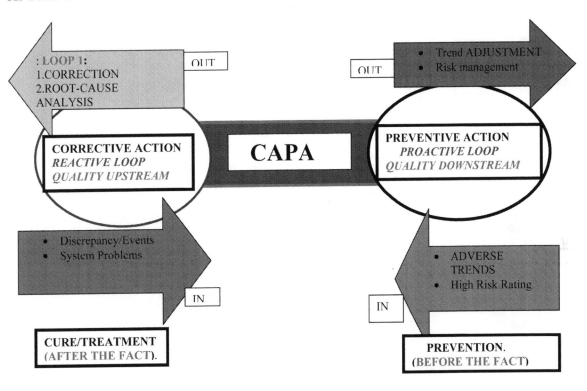

In the corrective loop, discrepancies (non-conformances, deviations, and events) are resolved through corrections and corrective action requests. In the preventive loop, adverse trends are adjusted through preventive action requests. Adverse trends that are not addressed in the preventive loop show up as problems to be investigated in the corrective loop. Resources (money, time, people, equipment, material) spent on the preventive loop go towards lowering the cost of poor quality that accompanies the reactive loop. In essence, prevention is better than cure. Efficient organizations spend less time putting out fires (in the ***reactive mode***); they spend time looking over the horizon for potential problems and situations that may lead to future problems if not addressed.

B. SYSTEM LAYOUT:

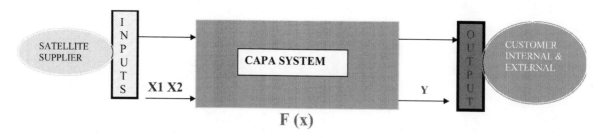

$$F(x)$$

The system can be looked at as ADDING VALUE to inputs X1 and X2 to produce outputs Y. There are two input streams, or loops, that feed the CAPA system:

(I) The internal loop feedback loop

(ii) The external loop feedback loop

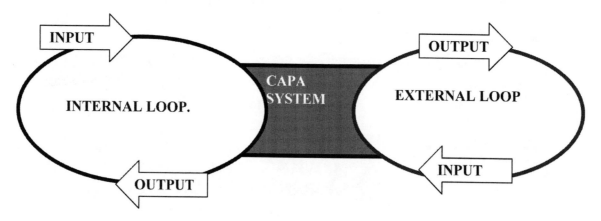

1. Internal loop: Primary inputs for this loop include:

- In-house audit findings
- Statistical process control charts
- Cost of quality (scrap, re-work, reject)
- Process control indices
- Test reports
- Incoming product reports
- In-process inspection
- Change control records
- Calibration records
- Equipment maintenance records
- Management review feedback
- Facilities environmental control records

2. External loop: Primary inputs for this loop include:

- Customer complaint records
- Warranties and concessions
- External audit findings: FDA 483s, warning letters, or ISO findings
- Customer returns records
- Field service reports

- Legal claims
- Product warranties
- MDR
- Product recalls

Analysis of primary inputs (quality records) leads to the generation of secondary inputs (X2) for the system: Corrective Action Requests (CARs), Preventive Action requests (PARs), Deviation Requests, Variance Requests, or Engineering Change Orders.

CARs are generated when analysis of quality records indicates the presence of any of the following:

- Unplanned deviations
- Non-conformances
- Discrepancies
- Complaints
- Unusual events

Preventive Action Requests (PARs), on the other hand, are secondary inputs for the proactive loop—the loop that proactively seeks to prevent future problems from happening. It utilizes any of the following:

- Statistical trends (run charts and Paretto charts)
- Risk analysis data (DFMEA and PFMEA, etc)
- Inherent variation
- Process control charts
- Annual product review (APR)
- Management review (quality metrics data and trends)
- Change requests
- Variance requests
- Engineering change requests
- Process capability indices (CpK and Cp)

The relationship between the output of the system and the inputs can be represented by the equation $Y=F(X2)$. Y results when F adds value to X. In this case, X2 represents all the CARs and PARs that come into the system. F represents the entire set of processes in all phases of CAPA from the discovery phase to the closure phase. CAPA system outputs include the following:

- Closure reports
- Management review reports
- Validation reports
- Escalation reports
- Investigation reports
- Effectiveness reports
- Status reports
- Change requests

- Root cause analysis report

This list is not carved in stone. What you choose as your output and primary input for your system is entirely up to you and the needs of the organization. It is, however, recommended that the source of the inputs be the conformance triangle: product, process, and the quality management system (QMS). A Corrective Action Request, or CAR, and a Preventive Action Request should have the following critical to quality attributes:

- Unique number
- Origin/department/organization
- Initiator's name or functional role
- Date initiated
- Ownership/responsible party

- Occurrence level (first or recurrence)
- The problem, or potential problem, source: product, process, or QMS

CORRECTIVE ACTION/PREVENTIVE ACTION REQUEST FORM.

CORRECTIVE/PREVENTIVE ACTION REQUEST		
CAR #	PAR#	DATE:
CATEGORY:☐ PRODUCT☐ PROCESS ☐ QMS.		
PROBLEM or POTENTIAL PROBLEM DESCRIPTION:		
DEPARTMENT:	OWNER:	
ACTION REQUESTED:		
INITIATOR: DEPARTMENT:	SIGNATURES: 1. Department 2. Quality	
System Admin: Date received:		

CHAPTER 3:
SATELLITE SUPPLIERS

All quality systems have some quality subsystems. The subsystems comprise satellite supplier systems to CAPA. These should be unique to your particular quality management system.

The first step in designing a CAPA system is the identification of the key suppliers to the system. At a high level, three suppliers of deviations, events, discrepancies, variances, and non-conformances exist. They make what is commonly referred to as the conformance triangle.

A. SUPPLIERS LAY OUT: HIGH LEVEL

1. PRODUCT/SERVICE

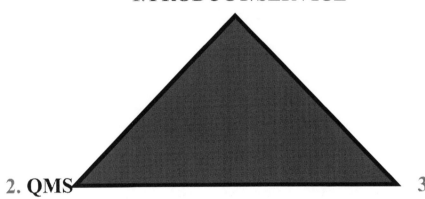

2. QMS   3. PROCESSES

The quality management system (QMS) comprises interrelated processes, which in turn produce products and services marketed by the organization to external customers.

At a system level, a CAPA subsystem should have at minimum the following satellite supplier subsystems:
- Supplier management
- Equipment and facilities control
- Production and process control
- Audit system
- Cost of quality
- Laboratory control system
- Customer management system
- Non-conformance material system
- Design control

- Document control
- Change control
- Management review

B. SATELLITE SUPPLIERS AND MANAGEMENT REVIEW LAYOUT

This is a representation of information flow between satellite supplier subsystems and the CAPA subsystem for any cGMP organization.

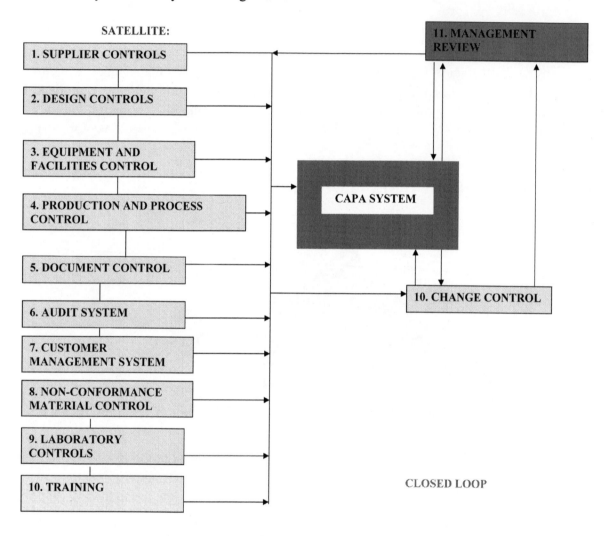

Each satellite supplier subsystem provides primary inputs in the form of quality reports (X1). Review of quality reports leads to the generation of secondary inputs to the CAPA system (X2): Corrective Action Requests (CARs) or Preventive Action Requests (PARs).

SATELLITE SUPPLIER subsystem: Customer management system

This subsystem feeds the CAPA system with the following primary inputs:

- Customer complaints records
- Returned goods records
- Service record
- Field actions record
- Adverse events records
- Product failure reports
- Customer feedback
- Concessions records
- Legal claims
- Product warranties
- Product performance records
- Supplier Corrective Action Requests (SCARs)

SATELLITE SUPPLIER subsystem: Production and process control

This subsystem feeds the CAPA system with the following primary inputs:

- In-process yield/defect records
- Inventory/quarantine product records
- Corrective maintenance (equipment down-time) records
- Statistical process control charts
- Document control records
- Training records
- Process validation records
- Change requests
- Variance requests
- Process run charts
- Process record review

SATELLITE SUPPLIER subsystem: Facilities and Equipment control

Provide the following primary inputs:

- Calibration and tolerance records
- Equipment preventive maintenance records
- Environmental monitoring records
- Facility maintenance records
- Equipment down-time records
- Equipment validation records
- Facility layout
- Facility protocols

SATELLITE SUPPLIER subsystem: Audit System

This subsystem provides the following primary inputs:

- Internal audit finding records
- External audit finding records (FDA 183s and ISO inspector findings)
- Quality system indicator trends

SATELLITE SUPPLIER subsystem: Supplier Management
- Supplier performance report
- Incoming reject report
- Supplier audit reports
- Supplier qualification report
- Supplier non-conformance report
- Material non-conformance report

SATELLITE SUPPLIER SUBSYSTEMS FOR SPECIFED INDUSTRIES

1. Medical Device industry

For the medical device industry, satellite supplier's subsystems to the CAPA subsystem should include all the quality subsystems outlined in 21CFR 820.5. The final list, however, should depend on your needs, your quality management system, and your infrastructure. Key satellite quality supplier subsystems:

Subpart B - THE QUALITY SYSTEM
- ❑ 820.20 Management responsibility
- ❑ 820.22 Quality audits
- ❑ 820.25 Personnel

SATELLLITE SUPPLIER: Subpart C
- ❑ 820.30 Design controls

SATELLITE SUPPLIER: Subpart D
- ❑ 820.40 Document controls

SATELLITE SUPPLIER: Subpart E
- ❑ 820.50 Purchasing controls

SATELLITE SUPPLIER: Subpart F
- ❑ 820.60 Identification and traceability

SATELLITE SUPPLIER Subpart G: Production and process control

820.70 Production and process control
- ❑ 820.72 Inspection, measuring, and test equipment
- ❑ 820.75 Process validation

SATELLITE SUPPLIER Subpart H: Acceptance activities
- ❑ 820.80 Receiving, in-process and finished device acceptance

SATELLITE SUPPLIER Subpart I: Non-conforming products.
- ❑ 820.90 Control of non-conforming products

SATELLITE SUPPLIER Subpart L: Storage and distribution
- 820.150 Storage
- 820.160 Distribution

SATELLITE SUPPLIER Subpart M: Records
- 820.181 Device master record
- 820.184 Device history record
- 820.186 Quality system record

- ❑ 820.198 Complaint files
- ❑ 820.200 Servicing records

SATELLITE SUPPLIER Subpart O: Statistical techniques
- ❑ 820.250 Process capability/product characteristic, adverse trend development statistical data.

Each satellite supplier sub systems should provide primary inputs to the CAPA system in the form of quality records, analysis of which should result in the generation of CARs, PARs, deviation requests, variance requests, or engineering change orders.

2. BIOLOGICS/BLOOD BANKING AND TRANSFUSION SERVICES

BLOOD AND BLOOD COMPONENTS:
Satellite suppliers to the CAPA system for biologics include, but are not limited to, the following:

SATELLITE SUPPLIER Subpart B: Organization and personnel
- 606.20 Personnel

SATELLITE SUPPLIER Subpart C: Plant and facilities
606.40 Plant and facilities

SATELLITE SUPPLIER Subpart D: Equipment
- 606.60 Equipment
- 606.65 Supplies and reagents

SATELLITE SUPPLIER Subpart F: Production and process controls
- 606.100 Standard operating procedures
- 606.110 Plateletpheresis, leukapheresis, and plasmapheresis

SATELLITE SUPPLIER Subpart G: Finished product control
- 606.120 Labeling

SATELLITE SUPPLIER Subpart H: Laboratory controls
- 606.140 Laboratory controls
- 606.151 Compatibility testing

SATELLITE SUPPLIER Subpart I: Records and reports
- 606.165 Distributions and receipt
- 606.170 Adverse reaction files
- 606.171 Reporting of product deviations by licensed manufactures, unlicensed registered blood establishments, and transfusion services.

It should be noted that this list is by no means final. The list of suppliers to your system should include what the organization deems critical to quality parameters for its processes, products, and quality management system.

SATELLITE SUPPLIERS FROM PART 640: HUMAN BLOOD AND BLOOD PRODUCT DERIVATIVE:

SATELLITE SUPPLIER SUBSYSTEM Subpart A: Standards for human blood and blood products
- 640.3 Donor suitability
- 640.4 Collection of blood
- 640.5 Testing of blood
- 640.6 Modification of whole blood

SATELLITE SUPPLIER SUBSYSTEM Subpart B: Red blood cells
- 640.12 Donor suitability
- 640.13 Collection
- 640.14 Testing
- 640.16 Processing
- 640.17 Modification for specific products

SATELLITE SUPPLIER SUBSYSTEM Subpart C: Platelets
- Donor suitability
- 640.23 Testing
- 640.24 Processing

Subparts D, F, G, H, and I.

The above satellite quality-subsystems should provide, at a minimum, the following primary inputs (X1) to your CAPA system:
- Donor suitability records
- Collection records
- Process records
- Compatibility records
- Laboratory records
- Adverse reaction records
- Look-back records
- Distribution records
- Storage records
- Management review records
- Personnel records
- Critical equipment records
- Document control records
- Computer records

This is a limited list. The total number of primary inputs will be unique to your quality management system and what your organization classifies as critical control points in your QMS.

3. DRUGS AND PHAMACEUTICALS

Satellite supplier subsystem to your CAPA subsystem should include the following:

SATELLITE SUPPLIER SUBSYSTEM Subpart B: Organization and personnel

- 211.22 Responsibilities of quality control unit
- 211.25 Personnel qualifications
- 211.28 Personnel responsibilities

SATELLITE SUPPLIER SUBSYSTEM Subpart C: Buildings and Facilities

- 211.42 Design and construction features
- 211.44 Lighting
- 211.48 Ventilation, air filtration, air heating and cooling
- 211.48 Plumbing
- 211.50 Sewage and refuse
- 211.56 Sanitation
- 211.58 Maintenance

SATELLITE SUPPLIER SUBSYSTEM Subpart D: Equipment

- 211.63 Equipment design, size, and location
- 211.67 Equipment cleaning and maintenance
- 211.68 Automatic, mechanical, and electronic equipment

SATELLITE SUPPLIER SUBSYSTEM Subpart E: Control of components and drug product containers and closures

- 211.82 Receipt and storage of untested components, drug product containers, and closures
- 211.84 Testing and approval or rejection of components, drug product containers, and closures
- 211.87 Retesting of approved components, drug product containers and closures
- 211.89 Rejected components, drug product containers, and closures

SATELLITE SUPPLIER SUBSYSTEM Subpart F: Production and process control

- 211.100 Written procedures; deviation: planned and unplanned
- 211.103 Calculation of yield
- 211.105 Equipment identification
- 211.110 Sampling and testing of in-process material and drug products
- 211.113 Control of microbiological contamination
- 211.115 Reprocessing/re-work

SATELLITE SUPPLIER-SUBSYSTEM Subpart G: Packaging and labeling

- 211.122 Materials examination and usage criteria
- 211.125 Labeling issuance
- 211.130 Packaging and labeling operations
- 211.134 Drug product inspection

SATELLITE SUPPLIER SUBSYSTEM Subpart H: Holding and distribution
- Warehousing procedures
- 211.150 Distribution procedures

SATELLITE SUPPLIER SUBSYSTEM Subpart I: Laboratory controls
- 211.165 Testing and release for distribution
- 211.165 Stability testing

SATELLITE SUPPLIER SUBSYSTEM Subpart J: Records and reports
- 211.182 Equipment cleaning and use log
- 211.184 Component, drug product container, closure, and labeling records
- 211.186 Master production and control records
- 211.188 Batch production and control records
- 211.192 Production record review
- 211.194 Laboratory records
- 211.196 Distribution records
- 211.198 Complaint files

SATELLITE SUPPLIER SUBSYSTEM Subpart K: Returned and salvaged drug products
- 211.204 Returned drug products
- 211.208 Drug product salvaging

It should be noted here that the list of satellite supplier subsystems above is not carved in stone. Placement of a quality subsystem on the supplier metrics depends on its strategic position and the role it plays in the overall quality management system.

PRIMARY INPUTS FOR THE PHARMACEUTICAL INDUSTRY:

- Personnel training records
- Facility maintenance records
- Equipment preventive maintenance records
- Equipment corrective maintenance records/logs
- Storage records
- Environmental records
- Process data
- Master production record
- Non-conformance material report
- Laboratory records

The complete list of inputs should be unique to your organization and your quality management system.

CHAPTER 4:
PRIMARY INPUTS

Quality records make up primary inputs to any CAPA subsystem. Records retain information after the fact. As the saying goes: "If it is not recorded, it didn't happen!" Analysis of quality records sets in motion secondary inputs: Corrective Action Requests (CARs), Preventive Action Requests (PARs), a Variance Request (VR), Engineering Change Request (ECR), or a Deviation Request (DR). For traceability purposes, each type of request should have its own unique numbering system. Any change request that affects product, process, or the QMS must be monitored through your CAPA information management system.

In general, quality records considered to be primary inputs to the CAPA system include, but are not limited to:
- Non-Conformance Material Reports (NCMR)
- Deviation Reports (DR)
- Monthly Trend Reports (MTR)
- Customer Complaint Report (CCR)
- Statistical Process Control charts (SPC)
- Trends charts (Paretto or run charts)
- Equipment Maintenance Reports (EMR)
- Equipment Calibration Record (ECR)
- Material Review Reports (MRR)
- Internal Audit Reports (IAR)
- External Audit Reports (483s and warning letters)
- Supplier assessment reports
- Employee training records
- Engineering change records
- Process capability charts (SQC charts)
- Laboratory control records
- Production yield records
- In-process data reports
- Distribution records
- Process and equipment validation reports
- Adverse events
- Environmental control records

Needless to say, the list of quality records can be overwhelming. However, it is the responsibility of the system designer to determine what the critical systems in the QMS are prior to establishing the supplier matrix.

For the preventive loop, inputs will also include the following:

- Engineering change requests/engineering change notes
- Deviation requests
- Variance requests
- Change requests
- Deviation requests
- Risk management records (PFMEA and DFMEA, or fault tree)
- Process run charts
- Process capability index data (CpK or Cp)

Trending of the first five is paramount. Trending points out inefficiencies in your processes and your quality management system as a whole.

For the medical device industry and ISO9001 certified organizations, critical satellite supplier subsystems that feed into the CAPA subsystem complement each other.

MEDICAL DEVICE INDUSTRY SATELLITE SUPPLIER SUBSYSTEMS

Supplier subsystems include: 820.20 Management responsibilities
Primary Input: Management review reports

Secondary inputs for the CAPA system from this quality subsystem include, but are not limited to:

1. 820.20(a) CARs and PARs related to events from the organization's quality policy
2. 820.20 (b) CARs and PARs, deviations, events, or non-conformance resulting from the organization structure, responsibility, authority, resource allocation, and management oversight of a quality management system.
3. 820.20(c) CARs and PARs, deviations, non-conformances, adverse trends, and events resulting from management review of the quality system performance data.
4. 820.20(d) CARs resulting from failures in quality planning, deviations from quality planning procedures, failures in meeting quality planning objectives, and failures in quality planning resource allocation.
5. 820.20 (e) CARs resulting from failures in following, implementing and monitoring effective quality system procedures and work instructions.

SATELLITE SUPPLIER SUBSYSTEM: 820.22 Quality audits

Primary Inputs: Internal and external audit reports
Secondary inputs from this quality subsystem include, but are not limited to:

6. CARs (Corrective Action Requests) resulting from internal quality management system audit findings.
7. CARs resulting from management reviews of internal and external audits.
8. CARs resulting from external audit citations and findings (FDA 483s or consent decree requirements)

SATELLITE SUPPLIER SUBSYSTEM: 820.25 Personnel

Primary Inputs: Training and personnel records.

Secondary inputs from this quality subsystem include the following:

1. CARs resulting from failure to meet training requirements
2. CARs resulting from insufficient personnel
3. CARs resulting from insufficient training programs
4. PARs resulting from adverse trends associated with personnel
5. CARs resulting from data obtained from training records

SATELLITE SUPPLIER SUBSYSTEM: 820.30 Design controls

Primary Inputs:

- Risk analysis data
- Deviation requests
- Variance/Engineering Change Requests (ECR)
- Design review records
- Validation records
- Master production record

Secondary inputs from this quality management subsystem should include:

1. 820.30(C) Deviations in the intended use of the end-user
2. 820.30 (b) CARs and PARs resulting from design reviews
3. 820.30 (b) PARs resulting from risk analysis data (e.g. DFMEA data).
4. 820.30(d) Deviations resulting from design output. This includes CARs and PARs related to packaging, labeling, and master production record review.
5. 820.30(e) CARs and PARs from design reviews.
6. 820.30 (f, g) CARs and PARs from discoveries made during validation and verification.
7. 820.30(h) CARS, PARs, and deviations resulting from design transfer (translation into production mode).
8. Variance requests
9. Deviation requests

SATELLITE SUPPLIER SUBSYSTEM: 820.50 Purchasing controls

This quality management subsystem controls the quality of purchased or otherwise products and service from internal and external suppliers of the organization. It provides control over the product, services, and suppliers. Final inputs to the CAPA system include the following:

PRIMARY INPUTS:

- Supplier performance record
- Supplier qualification data
- Supplier audit record
- Acceptance activity record

The secondary inputs include the following:
1. 820.50 (a) CARs and PARs from supplier evaluation and performance data
2. 820.50 (b) PARs and CARs from purchasing data review
3. Supplier deviations

SATELLITE SUPPLIER SUBSYSTEM: 820.70 Production and process control
Primary inputs:
- Production records
- Statistical process control charts
- Training records
- Document control records
- Process yield records
- Process capability records
- PFMEA records

This is, without a doubt, the largest supplier of secondary inputs into the CAPA system. These include, but are not limited to:

- 820.70(a) Deviations from standard operating procedures, deviations from process parameters, failure to meet workman standards, and failure to meet required specifications
- 820.70(b) CARs and PARS associated with process changes, SOP changes, tolerance changes, and methods
- 820.70(c) CARs and PARs associated with controlled elements in the production environment, environmental control methods, calibration intervals for the monitors, and changes in control limits
- 820.70(d) CARs and PARs associated with the health, cleanliness, and practices, training, and gowning protocol of production personnel
- 820.70 (e) CARs and PARs resulting from failure in contamination control, including cross-contamination of equipment, finished products, and environment
- 820.70 (f) Deviations, non-conformances, and discrepancies associated with workspace and building design
- 820.70 (g) Deviations, discrepancies, and non-conformances related to equipment maintenance schedules, equipment operating parameters, inspection cycles, and calibration cycles
- 820.70(h) adverse trends and problems associated with manufacturing materials
- 820.70 (I) CARs related to computer systems and software
- 820.72 CARs and PARs related to calibration cycles, calibration standards, and calibration tolerances
- 820.75 CARs and PARs from process performance data during process performance qualifications.

3. SATELLITE SUPPLIER SUBSYSTEM: PRODUCT and SERVICE
Primary inputs: Multiple
Secondary inputs from this section include the following:

❑ 820.120 CARs related to device labeling and specifications
❑ 820.130 CARs and PARs related to device packaging and distribution
❑ 820.140 CARs resulting from mix-ups, deterioration, contamination, and damage of product during handling
❑ 820.150 CARs and PARs related to storage parameters, storage conditions, and records
❑ 820.160 CARs related to distribution of the product
❑ 820.170 CARs and PARs related to product installation, test results, and servicing
❑ 820.90 CARs, and PARs resulting from non-conformity reviews (NMRB) and dispositions
❑ 820.198 CARs and PARs from analysis of customer complaint files
❑ 820.198 CARs and PARs resulting from reviews of service reports
❑ 820.40 Deviations from SOPs
❑ 820.198 CARs from customer complaint files

II. 21CFR Part 606: BLOOD AND BLOOD COMPONENTS

SATELLITE SUPPLIER SUBSYSTEM Subpart B: Organization and personnel
Secondary inputs: CARs and PARs on personnel and training records

SATELLITE SUPPLIER SUBSYSTEM: Subpart C: Plant and facilities
Secondary inputs: CARs and PARs on facility layout, process flow, ventilation system, and sewage system

SATELLITE SUPPLIER SUBSYSTEM Subpart D: Equipment
Secondary inputs: CARs and PARs on corrective and preventive maintenance, calibration, and equipment validation

SATELLITE SUPPLIER SUBSYSTEM Subpart F: Production and process controls
Secondary inputs: Deviations in standard operating procedures

SATELLITE SUPPLIER SUBSYSTEM Subpart H: Laboratory controls
Laboratory control records
Compatibility testing records

SATELLITE SUPPLIER SUBSYSTEM Subpart I: Records and reports
Production Records
Distribution and receipt reports
Adverse reaction files

PART 640: HUMAN BLOOD AND BLOOD PRODUCT DERIVATIVE SUPPLIERS

SATELLITE SUPPLIER SUBSYSTEM Subpart A: Standards for human blood and blood products

Primary Inputs:

    Donor suitability records

    Blood collection records

Testing of blood records

    Process Records

SATELLITE SUPPLIER SUBSYSTEM : Whole blood

1. Donor suitability records
2. Blood collection record
3. Blood testing record
4. Modification of whole blood records

SATELLITE SUPPLIER SUBSYSTEM Subpart B: Red blood cells

1. Donor suitability records
2. Collection records
3. Testing record
4. Processing record
5. Modification for specific products

SATELLITE SUPPLIER SUBSYSTEM Subpart C: Platelets

Donor suitability record

Testing records

Processing records

SATELLITE SUPPLIER SUBSYSTEMS: Subparts D, F, G, H, and I

PRIMARY INPUTS:

    A partial list of primary inputs to a CAPA system for blood banking and blood components manufacturers includes the following:

- Personnel/training records
- Review of standard operating procedures
- Errors in labeling control
- Annual process record review
- Distribution record review
- Adverse reaction records
- Equipment calibration record review
- Laboratory control review
- Facility layout and production process flow review
- Compatibility testing records
- Donor records
- Process records
- Storage and distribution records

- Compatibility records
- Quality control records
- Biological product deviations

The list is by no means exhaustive. The list of suppliers who end up on your supplier metrics depends on the critical control points (CCPs) in your quality management system.

III. DRUGS AND PHAMACEUTICALS

Suppliers to the CAPA system should include the following:

SATELLITE SUPPLIER SUBSYSTEM Subpart B: Organization and personnel

- 211.22 Responsibilities of quality control unit
- 211.25 Personnel qualifications
- 211.28 Personnel responsibilities

SATELLITE SUPPLIER SUBSYSTEM Subpart C: Buildings and facilities

These include the following:

- 211.42 Design and construction features
- 211.44 Lighting
- 211.48 Ventilation, air filtration, air heating and cooling
- 211.48 Plumbing
- 211.50 Sewage and refuse
- 211.56 Sanitation
- 211.58 Maintenance

SATELLITE SUPPLIER SUBSYSTEM Subpart D: Equipment

- 211.63 Equipment design, size, and location
- 211.67 Equipment cleaning and maintenance
- 211.68 Automatic, mechanical, and electronic equipment

SATELLITE SUPPLIER SUBSYSTEM Subpart E: Control of components and drug product containers and closures

- 211.82 Receipt and storage of untested components, drug product containers, and closures
- 211.84 Testing and approval or rejection of components, drug product containers, and closures
- 211.87 Retesting of approved components, drug product containers and closures
- 211.89 Rejected components, drug product containers, and closures

SATELLITE SUPPLIER SUBSYSTEM Subpart F: Production and process control

- 211.100 Written procedures; deviation
- 211.103 Calculation of yield
- 211.105 Equipment identification
- 211.110 Sampling and testing of in-process material and drug products

- 211.113 Control of microbiological contamination
- 211.115 Reprocessing/re-work

SATELLITE SUPPLIER SUBSYSTEM Subpart G: Packaging and labeling
- 211.122 Materials examination and usage criteria
- 211.125 Labeling issuance
- 211.130 Packaging and labeling operations
- 211.134 Drug product inspection

SATELLITE SUPPLIER SUBSYSTEM Subpart H: Holding and distribution
- Warehousing procedures, and distributions
- 211.150 Distribution procedures and deviations

SATELLITE SUPPLIER SUBSYSTEM Subpart I: Laboratory controls
211.165 Testing and release for distribution

SATELLITE SUPPLIER SUBSYSTEM Subpart K: Returned and salvaged drug products
211.204 Returned drug products

It should be noted here that the list of supplier subsystems above is not carved in stone. Placement of a quality subsystem on the supplier matrix depends on its strategic position among the systems that accomplish the organization's mission and objectives.

PHARMACEUTICAL INDUSTRY

SATELLITE SUPPLIER SUBSYSTEM Subpart J: Records and reports
This section lists primary inputs that feed the CAPA subsystem. They include, but are not limited to, the following:
- 211.182 Equipment cleaning and usage log
- 211.184 Component, drug product container, closure, and labeling records
- 211.186 Master production and control records
- 211.188 Batch production records
- 211.192 Production record review
- 211.194 Laboratory records
- 211.196 Distribution records
- 211.198 Customer complaint files

Others primary inputs include the following:

- 211.25 Training record review
- 211.28 Production protocol review
- 211.68 Calibration record
- 211.10 In-process data review

- 211.180 Complaints, recall, returned product, and salvage review
- 211.122 Receiving, labeling, and shipping records
- 211.42 Reviews of workflows and facility maintenance records
- 211.67 Review of equipment preventive maintenance records and logs
- 211.89 Reject report review
- 211.160 Lab control data
- 211.165 Quality performance data review
- 211.204 Returned product record review
- 211.103 Yield data review
- 211.208 Product salvage, re-work, and disposition record review

SATELLITE SUPPLIER SUBSYSTEM:
Subpart K-Returned and salvaged Drug products
- 211.204 Returned drug products, and Product disposition Record.

Again it should be noted that: the list of supplier subsystems above is not carved in stone. Placement of a quality subsystem on the supplier metrics depends on its strategic position as a critical control point in the quality management system and its role in accomplishing the organization's mission and objectives.

The supplier metrics should be representative of the compliance triangle:
- Processes that accomplish the mission
- Quality management system that manages how tasks are accomplished
- Product/service that the entire system produces for the organization's internal and external customers

CHAPTER 5:
SYSTEM MATRIX

The next step is to establish an input/supplier matrix. The matrix should answer the following questions:

Establishing the matrix accomplishes a specific regulatory requirement:
820.100 (a) (1) "An identified data source."

The matrix should address the following:
1. What to measure: Establish health indicators for each supplier satellite subsystem and its key processes.

2. Where to measure it: Establish a data collection point and primary inputs to be used in data analysis for specified suppliers and processes.

3. When to measure it: Establish the frequency for data analysis. Some organizations set up quarterly meetings for representatives from various functional groups, including process engineering and quality engineering, to review health indicators. Some organizations use management review meetings to accomplish this.

4. Who to measure it: Assign ownership. Whoever is assigned to accomplish this task should be familiar with the quality tool used. A person assigned to monitor process variability, for example, should be able to interpret SPC charts. A person measuring defects per million should be familiar with six sigma computations.

5. How to measure it: Select appropriate quality tools for data capture and analysis. Different parameters call for different measurement tools. Please choose the right tool, statistical or otherwise, for the given health indicator.

A. SUPPLIER MATRIX:

SATELLITE SUBSYSTEM (WHERE?)	QUALITY INDICATOR (WHAT?)	PRIMARY INPUT (WHAT?)	QUALITY TOOL (HOW?)	OWNERSHIP (WHO?)	FREQUENCY (WHEN?)	CFR REF.	OTHER REQUIREMENTS
1. CUSTOMER MANAGEMENT	1. Customer Returns 2. Corrective Action Requests 3. Customer Retention 4. Concessions 5. Recalls	1. Complaint Record 2. Complaint Record 3. Customer Record 4. Customer Record 5. NCM record	1. Paretto chart 2. Run chart records 3. Paretto chart 4. Run chart 5. Paretto chart	1. QC MANAGER 2. Q E 3. Quality council 4. PE 5. MRB	1. MONTHLY TREND 2. EACH COMPLAINT	820.50	
2. PRODUCTION AND PROCESS CONTROL.	1. Process yield 2. Process rejects 3. Change Requests 4. Planned and unplanned deviations 5. Variation		1. Process data 2. SQC 3. Production records 4. Non-conformance reports	1. PROCESS ENGINEER 2. PRODUCTION MANAGER	1. DAILY 2. MONTHLY	820.70	
3.AUDIT SYSTEM	1. Quality indices 2..Non-conformance 3. Legal fines	1.Audit Reports 2.DATA	1. Internal audit reports 2. External audit reports	AUDITOR	1. QUARTERLY 2. BI-ANNUAL		
4. PERSONNEL	1. Skill level 2. Retention 3. Training			HR MANAGER			
5.CHANGE CONTROL	1. Change request per process		1. DOE	DIRECTOR CHANGE CONTROL			
6.FACILITIES AND EQUIPMENT MANAGEMENT	1. Tolerance 2. Down time 3. Calibration cycles 4. Particle count per cubic ft.		1. SPC 2. PARETTO 3. DOE 4. SQC	FACILITIES MANAGER			
7.MANAGEMENT REVIEW			1. PARETTO	VP QUALITY			
8.DOCUMENT CONTROL	1. Plannned Deviations		1. Frequency Distribution	MANAGER CHANGE CONTROL			

Next, develop a CAPA system customer matrix.

The matrix should answer the following questions:

1. What information does the system generate?

2. For whom is this information generated?

3. How often is this information generated?

4. What critical quality attribute must this information have?

Now you need to establish what the system puts out, which it is put out for, how many times this happens, and established ownership.

B.CUSTOMER MATRIX

OUTPUT	CRITICAL TO QUALITY	CUSTOMER	FREQUENCY	OWNERSHIP
1. Investigation Report	Root cause	QC Unit head	Per incident	INVESTIGATIVE TEAM LEADER
2. Validation Report	Repeatability	QC Unit head	Per incident	ENGINEERING
3. Escalation report	Time	Site manager	Monthly	CAPA ADMIN
4. Change requests	Verification	Change control	Per Request	DEPARTMENTS
5. Management Review report	1. Disposition 2. Resource allocation	Process owners	Per Meeting	DIRECTOR QUALITY
6. Risk Assessment Report	1. RPN number 2. Trend	QC Unit head	Per incident	QUALITY UNIT
7. Closure Report	Signatures	QC Unit head CAPA Administrator	Per investigation	QUALITY UNITY
8. Deviation Requests	SOP	Document control	Per request	QUALITY UNIT
9. PROGRESS REPORT	1. Time 2.Measure of success	X	X	X
10. VALIDATION REPORT	X	X	X	X
11. QUARTERLY REPORTS	TRENDS	X	X	X
12. CONCESSION REPORT	PRODUCT DESPOSITION	INVENTORY CONTROL	PER INCIDENT	MRB

The two matrices should accomplish three things:
- Traceability
- Ownership
- Accountability

The customer matrix should have at a minimum eight customers/end users, namely:
1. A management representative with authority
2. Head of the QA function
3. Quality control function
4. Change control
5. Process engineering
6. External customers of the organization
7. Document control
8. Quality assurance function
9. Regulatory affairs
10. Manufacturing
11. CAPA administrator

The matrix provides a list of the end users of the system and the product they get from it, mostly QMS improvement information in the form of reports.

Third, establish a priority matrix for your problems and potential problems. Problems should be ranked and solved based on the risk posed to the process, product, or quality management system. The degree of action taken and resources allocated to the problem or potential problem should also depend on the magnitude of the problem and risk posed by doing nothing.

HOW DO YOU DECIDE WHAT PROBLEMS OR POTENTIAL PROBLEMS TO WORK ON?

C. PRIORITY MATRIX

CATEGORY	DEFINITION	INVESTIGATION DURATION	PRIORITY CODE	ESCALATION CRITARIA
1. Agent and important	(a) Events affecting product, process, customers, and the quality management system. (b) Needs containment action (c) Has system-wide implications (c) Has the potential for legal ramifications (d) Affects our profit margin	As soon as it is discovered	5 (MAJOR)	To VP quality if not resolved within 48 hours
2. Agent	(a) Affects production and quality of the product; may need containment/ recall or quarantine (b) May need MRB decision (c) Affects the bottom line of the organization	Within 24 hours	4	To VP Quality if not resolved within a week
3. Important	(a) Adverse trend exist (b) Has the potential to affect process, product, and end user (c) Has the potential to cut into the bottom line	Within 48 hours	3	To QA manager and QE if the trend persists after resolution
4. Needs to be done	A trend is developing	Within a week	2	To process engineering manager if not attempted in two weeks
5. Would be a good thing to do to improve the QMS	Process improvement	Within 2 weeks	1 (MINOR)	To VP quality if not attempted in two weeks

The problem resolution matrix establishes the order in which problems and potential problems in the CAPA system are handled. Problems coded 5 have higher priority. Those rated 1 are of least priority in the order of things. The matrix you come up with should be unique to your organization.

CHAPTER 6:
DISCOVERY VEHICLES

How do you find problems and potential problems?

Another important aspect of the discovery phase of the CAPA system is laying out how problems and potential problems in your quality management system are found and locked into the system. This should be done proactively. There are several discovery vehicles that can be used in a CAPA system. They include the following:

- Process audits
- External audits (ISO and FDA)
- Internal audits
- Management review
- Customer audits
- Batch reviews
- Quarterly quality record reviews
- Personnel review
- Supplier audits
- Annual quality record reviews

This list is not carved in stone. Different organizations rely on different discovery vehicles. Choose discovery vehicles that work for your organization. The important point is that they are documented.

DISCOVERY VEHICLES AND DATA COLLECTION FREQUENCY

DISCOVERY VEHICLE	FREQUENCY	OWNERSHIP	PRIMARY INPUT
1. Process Auditing	1. DAILY	1. PROCESS ENG.	
2. External Auditing			1. PROCESS RECORDS
3. Internal Auditing	2. BI-ANNUAL	2. QA	2. AUDIT REPORT
			3. AUDIT REPORT
4. Management Review	3. ANNUALY	3. QA	
5. Customer Audits	5. MONTHLY	5. QE	5. AUDIT FINDING REPORT
6. Batch Review	4. WEEKLY	4. MANAGEMENT	4. MANAGEMENT REPORT
7. Personnel	7. N/A	7. PERSONNEL	7. Discrepancy report
8. Annual Quality Review	8. ANNUAL	6. PROCESS ENG.	8. Annual quality report
9. Incoming Acceptance Activities	6. WEEKY	8. QA	6. Batch records
	9. DAILY		9. Reject report
		9. Receiving	
10. Final Inspection	10. Daily		10. Yield report
		10. QA	

CHAPTER 7:
REQUIREMENTS

A CAPA system must meet at a minimum THREE sets of requirements:
1. Business requirements
2. Regulatory requirements
3. Information management system requirements

1. BUSINESS REQUIREMENTS:

Most businesses follow the ISO business requirements for a Corrective Action/Preventive Action (CAPA) subsystem. These complement CAPA requirements in 21CFR820.100 (J).

A. ISO 9001:2000 (E) REQUIREMENTS:

The ISO 9001:2000 (E) quality management system requires organizations to continuously improve the quality management system's effectiveness through:
- Audit results
- Data analysis
- Corrective action and preventive actions
- Management review

The standard specifically calls for:
8.5.2 CORRECTIVE ACTION.

(I) Taking action to eliminate the cause of non-conformities in order to prevent RECURRENCE ("after the fact").
(II) Making sure that the corrective action taken is appropriate to the effects of the non-conformities encountered.

The section also calls for documented procedures for:
(a) Reviewing non-conformities
(b) Determining the cause of non-conformities
(c) Evaluation of the need for action to ensure the non-conformity does not happen again
(a) Determining and implementing action needed
(b) Maintaining records of the results of action taken
(c) Review of the corrective action taken

8.5.3 PREVENTIVE ACTION:

This section calls for the organization to determine action to eliminate the cause of potential non-conformities in order to prevent their OCCURRENCE ("before the fact"). It also calls for established, documented procedures to define requirements for the following:

- Determining potential non-conformities and their causes
- Evaluating the need for action to prevent occurrence of non-conformities
- Determining and implementing action needed
- Records of results of action taken
- Reviewing preventive action taken

The ISO requirements provide a framework for most business requirements. They provide a skeleton. It is up to the system designer to make those requirements specific and in line with the organization's mission, culture, and infrastructure.

B. ISO 9001 REQUIREMENTS

Section 4.14: CORRECTIVE AND PREVENTIVE ACTION

The section calls for a quality subsystem with both reactive and proactive modes for continuous process, product, and quality system improvement.

4.14.2 CORRECTIVE ACTION (CA): (reactive mode): Dealing with actual non-conformities.

Purpose: Investigation of existing product problems, quality problems, and process failure problems.

Requirements:
1. Effective handling of customer complaints and reports of product non-conformity.
2. The Investigation of the cause of non-conformities related to product, process, and quality system; documentation of the investigation.
3. Standard protocol for determining the corrective action needed to eliminate the cause of non-conformities.
4. Application of controls to ensure that corrective action is taken and is effective.
5. Process ownership ("who does what").
6. Definition of the process.
7. Effectiveness/measure of success.

4.14.3 PREVENTIVE ACTION (PA): (proactive mode): Dealing with clouds that may be gathering on the horizon; potential problems.

Purpose: Controls and investigates undesirable trends and patterns that point to potential future quality, process, and system problems.

REQUIREMENTS:

1. The ability to use information from processes, concessions, quality audit records, service reports, and customer complaints to detect, analyze, and eliminate potential causes of non-conformities.
2. Protocol for the determination of the need for preventive action.
3. Steps for initiation of preventive action.
4. Check for effectiveness.
5. Submission of relevant information on actions taken for management review.

Hybrids of these ISO requirements do exist for different industries. The American Association of Blood Banks has its own standards for corrective action and preventive action system for those in the blood banking and tissue business. These standards complement the ISO 9001 requirements:

AABB CAPA STANDARDS FOR BLOOD BANKS AND TRANSFUSION SERVICES

Section 9.0: Process Improvement through Corrective and Preventive Action

9.1 CORRECTIVE ACTION (CA):

This section calls for an established corrective action system which accomplishes the following:

9.1.1 Documents incidents, error, accident reports, non-conformance reports, and complaints

9.1.2 Investigates non-conformances related to blood, components, tissue, derivatives, critical materials, and services

9.1.3 Investigates customer complaints

9.1.4 Determines corrective action needed to eliminate incidents, errors, and accidents

9.1.5 Evaluates the effectiveness of the corrective action taken

9.2 PREVENTIVEACTION: (PA):

This section calls for an established preventive action system which accomplishes the following:

9.2.1 Reviews information from assessment results, proficiency testing results, quality control records, and complaints to detect and analyze potential causes of non-conformances

9.2.2 Determines steps needed to deal with potential problems requiring preventive action

9.2.3 Initiates preventive action and applies controls for effectiveness

1. BUSINESS REQUIREMENT MATRIX

Most organizations use ISO 9001:2000 quality management system requirements as their business requirements. These requirements are compatible with ISO 14001. A summary is provided below.

ISO 9001:2000(E)	SYSTEM BUSINESS REQUIREMENTS
4.1	➢ Establish, document, implement, maintain, and continuously improve the quality management system
4.2	➢ Standard procedures for process control and personnel competence
5.1	➢ Established quality policy, quality objectives, management review, and resource allocation
5.2	➢ Customer focus
5.3	➢ Commitment to meet customer requirements and continual process improvement
5.4.1	➢ Established, measurable quality objectives and commitment to continuous improvement
5.4.2	➢ Resource allocation for quality objectives and controlled changes.
5.5.2	➢ Defined functional roles
5.5.3	➢ Member of management team with responsibility to oversee the QMS FUNCTION
5.5.4	➢ EFFECTIVE INTERNAL QMS COMMUNICATION SYSTEM
5.5.5	➢ Documented quality manual.
5.5.6	➢ Document control through controlled quality records, revision levels, and version control
5.5.7	Documented procedures for the identification, storage, retrieval, protection, retention, and disposition of quality records
5.6.1	Management review of the QMS FOR EFFECTIVENESS
5.6.2	Review of audit results, customer input, process performance, and product conformance followed by corrective action, or preventive action
5.6.3	Management resource allocation for process, product and QMS improvement
6.1	Resource allocation for process improvement, and customer satisfaction
6.2.1	Personnel qualification
6.2.2	Training and competencies of QMS personnel
6.3	Facilities: workspace, equipment, hardware and supporting services
6.4	Environmental control: control of the physical factors affecting the work environment
7.1	Planning off realization: process validation
7.2.1	Determination of product requirements, customer requirements, and customer requirements
7.2.3	Established customer communication system: an established system through which the customer communicates with the organization
7.3.1	Design control, verification, validation, and team interface
7.3.2	Design inputs: functional, performance, regulatory, and legal
7.3.3	Design outputs: verifications against input requirements, and defined product characteristics
7.3.4	Design review to identify potential problems
7.3.5	Design verification: reconciliation of inputs and outputs

7.3.6	Design validation before product delivery
7.3.7	Control of design changes; approval of changes before implementation
7.4.1	Purchase control: supplier qualification
7.4.2	Purchasing: procedures, processes, and personnel requirements
7.4.3	Verification of purchased products
7.5.1	Operations control; production process control
7.5.2	Identification and traceability of product
7.5.5	Process validation
7.6	Control of measuring devices
8.0	Measurement, analysis and improvement

2. REGULATORY REQUIREMENTS

CAPA system requirements are defined in the medical device code of federal regulations. This CFR outlines a common-sense business approach to problem solving and deviation management. The requirements complement those set for corrective action and preventive action in the ISO 9001 quality management system. Here is a summary of the requirements:

It is recommended that the system designer develop a requirement matrix for each set of requirements. It is also recommended that the final system requirement matrix be a combination of the three sets of requirements: business, regulatory, and information system management requirements.

REGULATORY REQUIREMENTS MATRIX

21CFR 820.100 SUBPART J	CAPA SYSTEM REQULATORY REQUIREMENTS *THE SYSTEM MUST HAVE:*
1.820.100(a)	➤ Defined, documented and maintained procedures for implementing preventive and corrective action
2.820.100(a)(1)	➤ Identified quality data sources (matrix)
	➤ Processes for analysis of quality data, concessions, quality audits, SOPs, complaints, quality records, service records, returned products for potential causes of non-conforming products
	➤ The ability to use SPC to detect recurring problems
	➤ The ability to use quality data to solve quality problems that require corrective action
3.820.100(a)(2)	➤ An investigation process for causes of non-conformities related to products, processes, and the QMS
4.820.100(a)(3)	➤ Established method for root-cause analysis to identify actions needed to correct and prevent recurrence of non-conforming products and other quality problems
5.820.100(a)(4)	➤ A validation process for all corrective actions and preventive actions prior to implementation

6. 820.100(a)(5)	➤ The capability to document all implemented changes in methods and procedures to correct and prevent quality problems
8.820.100(a)(6)	➤ Timely dissemination of information related to quality problems to those responsible
9.820.100(a)(7)	➤ A closed loop with information forwarded to a person with authority for management review and resource allocation
820.100 (b)	➤ The ability to record and maintain *all* activities, tasks performed, and results obtained
	TRACEABILITY!

There are other inputs that go into the CAPA system for traceability purposes; these include the following:

- Variance requests (VR)
- Engineering change notes (ECNs)
- Deviation requests (DR)
- Change requests (CRs)

As a rule of thumb, any changes that affect processes, products, and the quality management system must be tracked through he CAPA system. An increase in change requests, deviation requests, or engineering change notes depicts inefficiencies and inherent variation in your processes.

3. INFORMATION MANAGEMENT REQUIREMENTS

It is imperative to have an information management system for your CAPA system, not only for traceability and accountability purposes, but also to have customer and supplier involvement in problem solving and quality improvement. For that reason, it is recommended that your information management system meet the following conditions:

(a) Be web-based. All that is needed is a web browser. Most computers are sold with this gizmo anyway.

(b) Not be client/server technology requiring application-specific software that requires configuration on client computers.

(c) Provide real-time information and analyses, to cut down on response time on critical situations like recalls, quarantine, and containment.

(b) Be part of your core information system, not a QA database.

(c) Work across all types of operating systems and platforms, including Windows, Mac, UNIX, Linux, Solaris and Palm.

(d) Offer easy configuration and customization of forms, fields, workflows, and security settings.

(e) Be easily integrated with other information systems already installed in your organization.

(f) Have bulletproof security with limited access to users and departments, such as thwarting repeated attempts to gain unauthorized access, and immediate notification to the system administrator of the threat.

(g) Allow for file attachments and storage

(h) Have a universal email integration capability.

(i) Allow for definitions for task escalation to management.

(j) Be 21 CFR Part 11 compliant. This part governs electronic records and electronic signatures:

- A secure time-stamped audit trail of all actions taken
- Application of signatures only by genuine owners
- Password protection
- Session time-out
- Lock-out upon failed login attempts
- Activity history
- Different authorization levels

(k) Have graphical statistical analysis capability

(l) Have reports and graph generation capability

INFORMATION MANAGEMENT REQUIREMENT MATRIX

	INFORMATION MANAGEMENT REQUIREMENTS
1.PART 11	➢ Time-stamped audit trail of all actions taken
	➢ Signatures by approved personnel
	➢ Password protection
	➢ Session time-out
	➢ Activity history log for traceability
	➢ Multi-authorization levels
2. END-USER	➢ Statistical analysis capability
	➢ Reports and graph generation capability
	➢ File attachment capability
	➢ Easy configuration
	➢ Ability to work across other operating systems
	➢ Ability to provide real-time information for users
	➢ Preferably web-based
	➢ Compatible with your current infrastructure

Once you have developed your three sets of requirements, it is recommended that you compile a whole system requirement map. This is done for requirement traceability purposes. As a system designer, you have to know if your system meets all the requirements, especially regulatory requirements. The best way to do this is to draft a requirement traceability matrix.

REQUIREMENT TRACEABILITY MATRIX

REQUIREMENT CLASS	REQUIREMENT DESCRIPTION	REQUIREMENT NUMBER	DOC. NUMBER	CUSTOMER	DOCUMENT DESCRIPTION
1. REGULATORY	(a) Established procedures	820.100(a)	QA0019	FDA, QUALITY MANAGER	STANDARD OPERATING PROCEDURES
	(b) Established data source	820.100(a)	PMQ 0023	FDA, ISO 9001	SUPPLIER MATRIX
	(c) Data analysis	820.100(a) 1	QA 611	ISO 9001	DISCOVERY VEHICLES
	(d) etc				
2. BUSINESS	(a) Continuous process improvement	MX----	QA----	VP QUALITY	
	(b) Customer focus	XC---	PC----	VP QUALITY	
	(c) etc.				
3. INFORMATION MANAGEMENT SYSTEM	(a) Part 11 Compliance	21 CFR part 11	IT 532	IT manager	POLICY ON Electronic signatures
	(b) etc				

■ CHAPTER 8:
HIGH-LEVEL MAPS

The next step in the design process is to come up with a high-level system overview: a general map of the entire system. Ask yourself five key questions:

1. When is corrective action or preventive action initiated?
2. What happens when a problem needs immediate attention?
3. How is the problem or potential problem resolved?
4. What is needed to resolve the problem or potential problem?
5. How do you test the success of your corrective or preventive action?
6. What happens when a potential problem, or problem, is not resolved in a timely manner, or when an old problem recurs?

POTENTIAL ANSWERS TO THE QUESTIONS ABOVE:

Here are potential answers to the questions above:
1. Upon discovery
2. It is contained
3. It is investigated
4. Execution of a plan
5. Through assessment
6. It is escalated.

Different people in different organizations may come up with different answers to these same questions. However, based on the answers above, the road map for the CAPA system is clear: It starts with discovery and ends with assessment. The sequence of events then becomes:

 1. Discovery   **2. Containment**
3. Investigation   **4. Execution**
5. Assesment   **7. Closure**
6. Escalation.

QUESTION: When do you escalate a problem to management?

ANSWER: You don't, unless you really have to. Problems have to be solved at the source. For that reason, escalation is never counted as a phase in CAPA, though it really should.

The sequence of events above is what is what is referred to as the high-level phases of the CAPA system. It should be noted also that escalation of a problem or potential problem can take place at any stage between the phases. The criteria for escalation vary from organization to organization. The most acceptable criterion for escalation of a problem or potential problem is recurrence of the same problem and the severity it poses to the product, service, process, or the quality management system. Problems are usually escalated for management intervention.

There are two types of high-level maps. Below are general examples of high-level maps for a CAPA system. In the first example, the phases through which work gets accomplished are left to the designer. Phase I could be discovery, phase II could be containment. Again, the choice is yours.

TYPES OF HIGH-LEVEL MAPS

Several types of high-level maps exist. The choice is yours. A high-level map accomplishes two things: first, it paints a picture of the path followed in the system. Second, it determines the number of processes and process steps in the system.

1. Type one:

Type one map is a functional map with no defined phases. It is generic in nature. The designer defines the phases on this map.

2. Type 2:

Type two maps are the most used, and are preferred by most designers because they are divided into distinct phases with distinct names and action items.

A.   TYPE ONE HIGH-LEVEL MAPS

In this high-level map, the criterion for escalation is whether the corrective action/preventive action passes effectiveness check or not. The criterion for escalation in most systems is the investigation cycle. The phases run parallel to each other. The actions are fluid and independent of the phase.

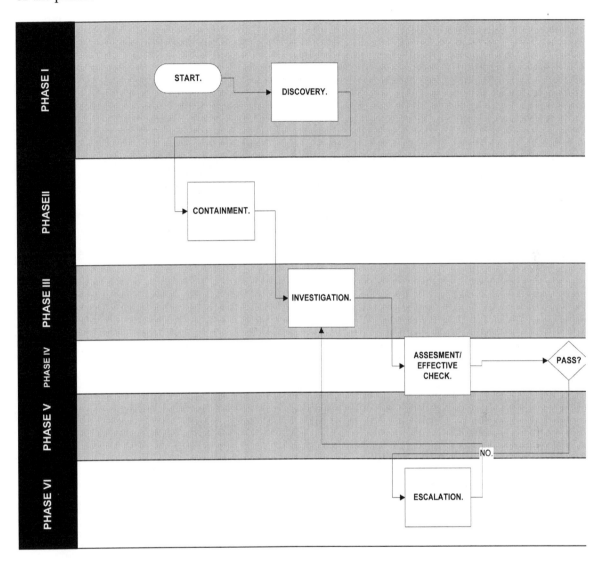

B. TYPE TWO HIGH LEVEL MAP

In the second example, processes through which tasks are accomplished are specified for each phase:

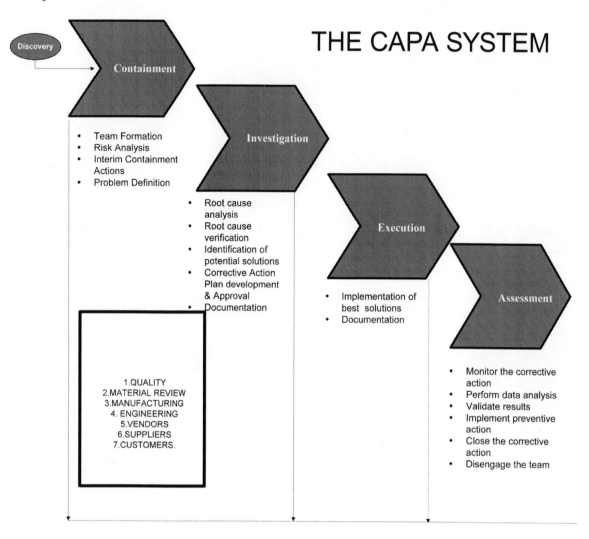

THE CAPA SYSTEM

Discovery

Containment
- Team Formation
- Risk Analysis
- Interim Containment Actions
- Problem Definition

Investigation
- Root cause analysis
- Root cause verification
- Identification of potential solutions
- Corrective Action Plan development & Approval
- Documentation

1.QUALITY
2.MATERIAL REVIEW
3.MANUFACTURING
4. ENGINEERING
5.VENDORS
6.SUPPLIERS
7.CUSTOMERS.

Execution
- Implementation of best solutions
- Documentation

Assessment
- Monitor the corrective action
- Perform data analysis
- Validate results
- Implement preventive action
- Close the corrective action
- Disengage the team

CHAPTER 9:
KEY PROCESSES

A CAPA subsystem should have a minimum of five high-level phases. They are as follows:

1. DISCOVERY

This phase encompasses processes and procedures for periodic analysis and review of product, process, and QMS data to develop actions to prevent occurrence or recurrence of problems and potential problems. There are key questions that need to be answered for each phase. For the discovery phase, the key questions are as follows:

How are problems and potential problems found? In other words, what are the discovery vehicles? Remember, one of the regulatory requirements for a CAPA subsystem is that the organization has to be actively looking for problems and potential problems.

For most organizations, ten major discovery vehicles exist:
- Internal system audits
- External system audits (FDA483s and warning letters)
- Process audits
- Product annual reviews
- Management review meetings
- Supplier audits
- Supplier review and qualification
- Customer management record reviews
- Production/batch record reviews
- Equipment management record review (corrective and preventive maintenance down time)
- Process and equipment calidation
- Risk management reviews
- Annual product reviews
- Non-conformance Material Review Board (NMRB)

These discovery vehicles are used in data analysis of all primary inputs (quality records); the output of the analysis is the secondary input into the system: Corrective Action Requests (CARs) or Preventive Action Requests (PARs).

Your list of discovery vehicles should be based on your culture, your mission, the complexity of your system, and your Quality Management System (the QMS of your organization).

The discovery phase should have a minimum of the following processes:
- Analysis of quality records

45

- Initiation of a CAR or PAR
- Approval of a PAR or CAR
- Priority assignment

Finally, develop a rough draft of workflows between departments during the discovery phase.

CAPA by default is a cross-functional system. It is imperative that this is taken in account while drafting your workflows.

INTER-DEPARTMENT WORK FLOW TYPE ONE

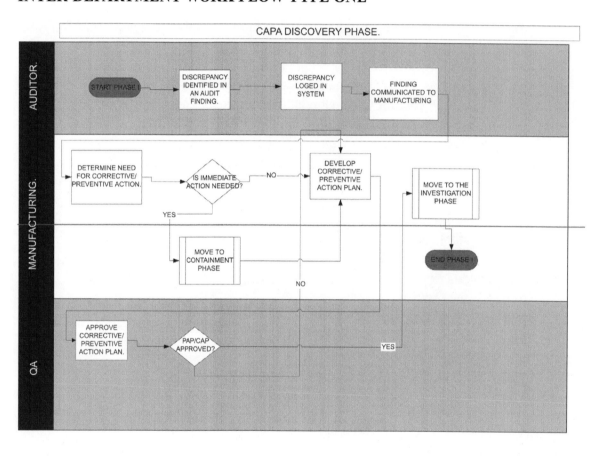

INTER-DEPARTMENT WORK FLOW TYPE TWO:

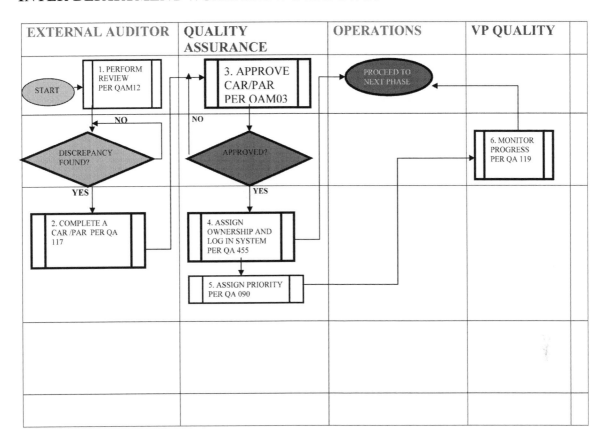

PHASE II: CONTAINMENT

The containment phase addresses agent problems and events. It also addresses potential problems that, if left unattended, may show up in the corrective loop with financial ramifications. The questions that drive this phase are as follows:

1. What is the problem or potential problem?
2. Is it agent and important?
3. What should we do to correct it while we look for a long-term solution?
4. Does it affect our mission?
5. What is the risk involved?
6. What is its effect on product, process, and quality management system?
    Examples here include:
    (a) Non-conforming products
    (b) Out of specification equipment
    (c) Returned products
    (d) Non-conforming material
    (e) Legal issues
    (f) Regulatory citation
    Action that may be taken to contain the problem may include:

- Stopping production
- Reworking the product
- Requesting an engineering change
- Quarantining the product
- Requesting a variance
- Requesting a deviation
- Recalling the product
  The key processes in this phase include the following:
  1. Problem definition
  2. Risk analysis
  3. Risk containment
  4. Evaluation of the effects of risk containment on product, process, and the quality management system

INTER-DEPARTMENT WORK FLOW TYPE ONE

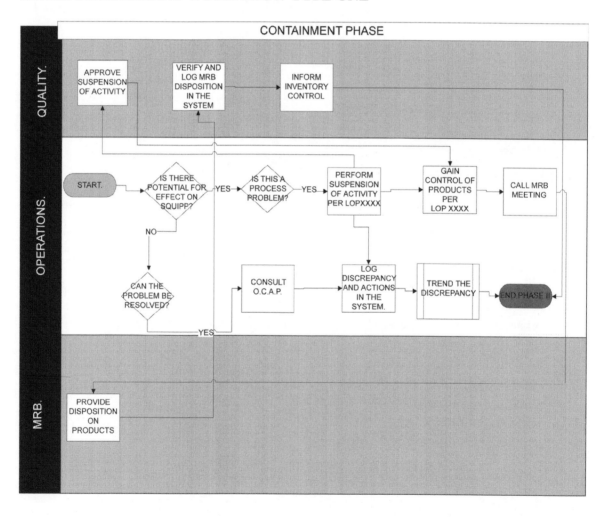

INTER-DEPARTMENT WORK FLOW TYPE TWO:

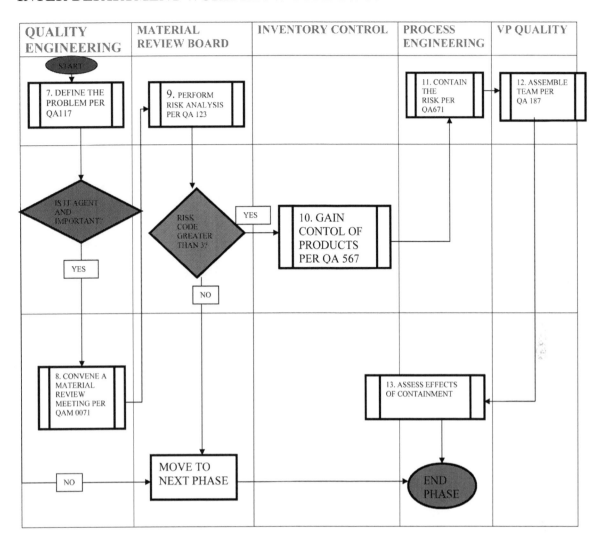

PHASE III: INVESTIGATION

This phase aims at getting to the root of the matter and the best way to resolve the problem or potential problem. It includes the following key processes:

- Root cause analysis
- Brainstorming for solutions
- Determination of best solution to the problem
- Development of corrective action/potential problem plan
- Approval of the plan
- Assessing the need for escalation

It should be noted that that this is a very important phase in the CAPA system. It is a phase that determines whether an issue should be escalated to upper management or not.

INTER-DEPARTMENT WORK FLOW TYPE ONE

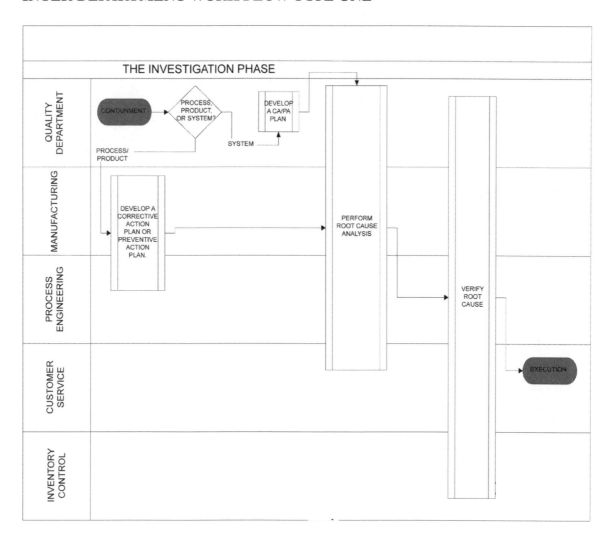

INTER-DEPARTMENT WORK FLOW TYPE TWO

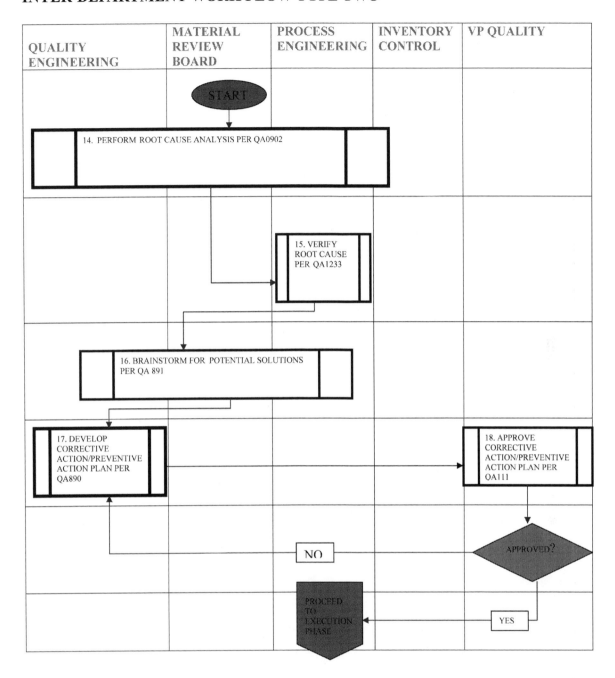

PHASE IV: EXECUTION

This phase aims at the implementation of best solutions to the problem or potential problem. Four processes exist. They are as follows:

- Data gathering
- Data analysis
- Effectiveness check
- Change request
- Implementation

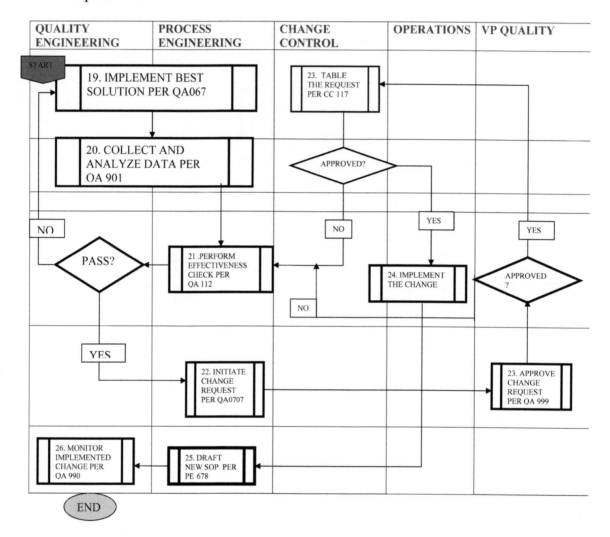

PHASE V: ASSESMENT

This phase involves:

- Analysis of results obtained
- Validation
- Closure or escalation

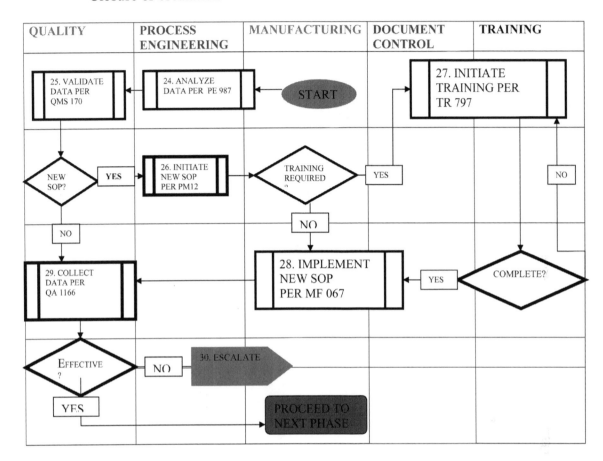

CHAPTER 10: DEPARTMENAL WORKFLOWS

The next task is to establish "who does what" in each phase of your system. Functional roles have to be established. Second-level cross-functional maps establish process ownership, an essential element in a CAPA system since, by default, a CAPA system is cross-functional.

The map also establishes processes and process steps. A clear distinction needs to be made between a process and a process step: A process, by definition, adds value to provided inputs to produce an output that is used by an end user, or customer. A process step, on the other hand, is exactly that: a step. Another distinction exists: On a process map, a process step is represented by a rectangle.

Diagram: 1
   PHASE: DISCOVERY
   PROCESS: 1. Corrective Action Initiation
   DOCUMENT: XXX 0100

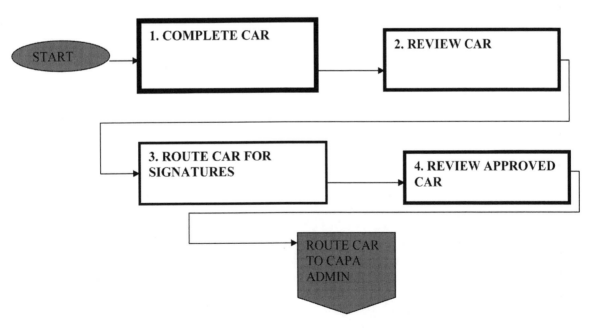

All processes have standard operating procedures (SOPs), third-level documents that are used in accomplishing tasks. Tasks are accomplished in steps, as shown above. The numbering of your work instructions should follow the format established by your document control system. For this reason, it is imperative to work with the document control group when you start drafting level two and level three documents.

Each CAPA phase should be broken down into its processes and then process steps. The number of processes and processes steps in each phase depends on the complexity of the system. However, you should audit your processes for steps that don't add value to the input.

One of the key processes in the discovery phase is the initiation of a Corrective Action Request. The initiation is a process that is accomplished by the use of third-level documents, also called work instructions or Standard Operating Procedures (SOPs). In the examples below and above, tasks are accomplished using a set of instructions in document XXX. The boxes in the process box represent steps that accomplish tasks leading to a completed Corrective Action Request, or CAR.

Diagram 2:
   PHASE: DISCOVERY
   PROCESS: Corrective Action Initiation
   DOCUMENT: XXX

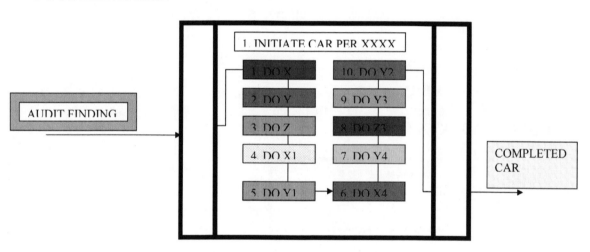

Here is an actual example of processes in a discovery phase and how work gets accomplished. There are two process owners: Quality and the External Auditor.

PHASE: DISCOVERY
VEHICLE: External Auditing

   PROCESSES:
   - Initiation of Corrective Action Request/Preventive Action Request
   - Logging CAR/PAR in the system
   - Categorizing CAR/PAR in the system
   - Assigning ownership
   - Routing the CAR

PART 1: INTERDEPARTMENT WORKFLOW: LEVEL 2

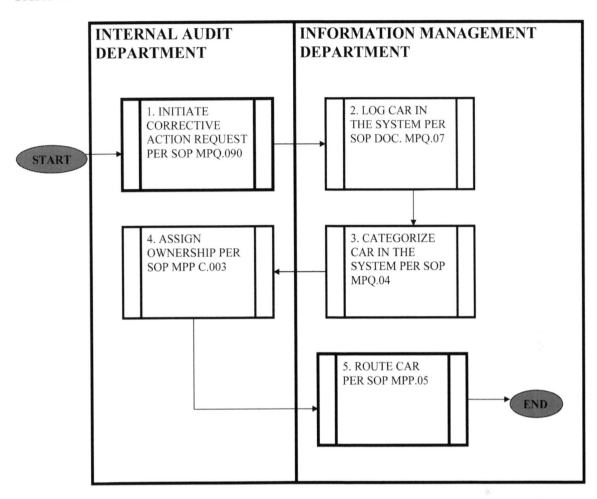

Note: each process is defined by its work instructions. Work instructions outline steps through which tasks are accomplished. They are numbered according to your document system.

LEVEL 3: TASK ACCOMPLISHMENT

Every phase has processes. Processes have process steps, which accomplish tasks. Set role players accomplish tasks. During discovery, for example, initiation of a CAR is a process that can be handled by several role players at task accomplishment level: the auditor from the quality department and a CAPA administrator from the information management department. Other teams from different departments or the same department may handle other processes that follow in the phase.

Here is the path to be followed. This should be very obvious to you by now:

1. PHASES:
"THE PATH
FORWARD"

CAPA phases

2. PROCESS:
WHAT
DEPARTMENT DOES
WHAT?

Processes per phase

3. TASKS:
WHO IS DOING WHAT
IN THOSE
DEPARTMENTS?

Tasks in each process

Roles

**4. WORK
INSTRUCTIONS:**
HOW IS IT BEING
DONE?

PHASE: DISCOVERY
PROCESS: CAR INITIATION: TASK LEVEL (LEVEL 3)

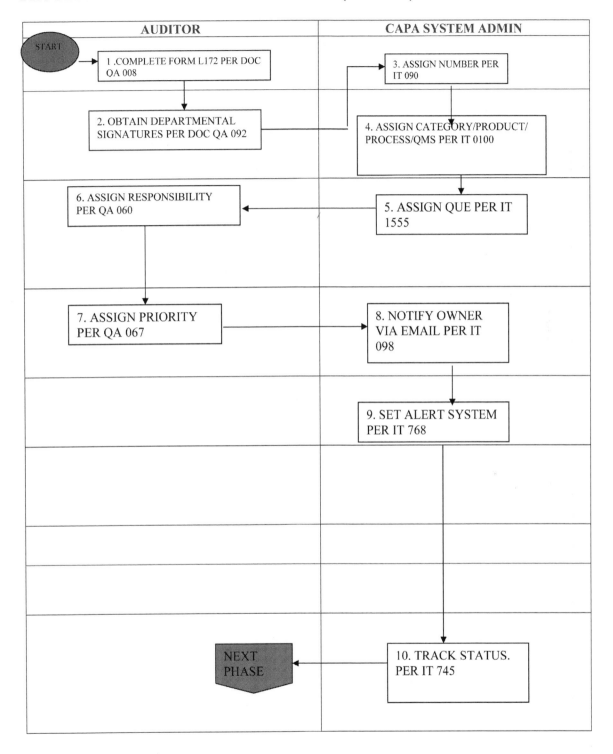

PHASE 2: CONTAINMENT

PROCESSES IN THE PHASE:
- Problem definition

- Determination of effect on product
- Product control
- Suspension of activities
- NMR disposition
- OCAP (Out-of-Control Action Plan)

DEPARTMENTAL WORKFLOW:

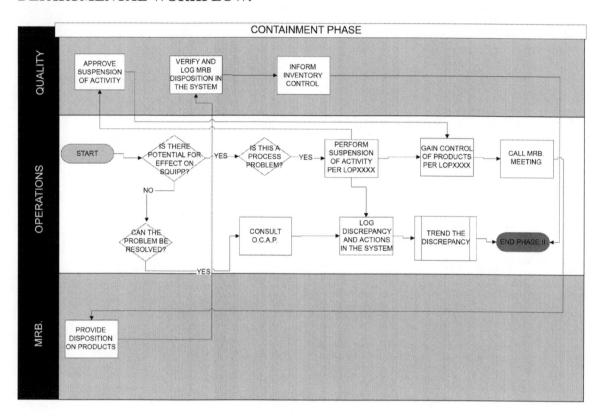

Note: trending discrepancies in the above process map is a process; hence, it should be accompanied by work instructions.

PHASE 3: INVESTIGATION
PROCESSES IN THE PHASE:

- Developing a corrective action plan or a preventive action plan
- Performing root-cause analysis
- Verifying root cause
- Management
- Resource allocation

Each of these processes accomplishes particular tasks using a set of work instructions. Your work instructions are level three documents. They are process work-steps that produce a particular output.

DEPARTMENTAL WORKFLOW

In the example given below, the development of a Corrective Action Request or Corrective Action Report is a process that cuts through two departments: process engineering and manufacturing. On the other hand, the root cause analysis process cuts across process engineering, quality, manufacturing, and customer service.

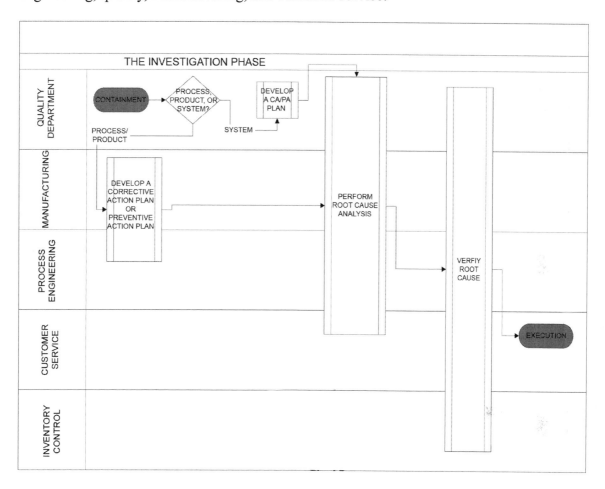

Note: Four cross-functional processes exist in the above map. They should be accompanied by individual work instructions for different work steps.

PHASE 3: EXECUTION

PROCESSES IN THE PHASE:
- Implementation of best solutions
- Monitoring of implemented solutions
- Collection of data
- Data analysis
- Validation of implemented solution
- Change reques

PHASE 4: CLOSURE
PROCESSES:
- Review by responsible person with authority
- QA assessment

Top management review

CHAPTER 11:
WORK INSTRUCTIONS

Third-level maps are work steps. They provide the sequence of events in a process. They outline how work gets done.)

Example:

PROCESS: Validation of corrective action
DOCUMENT: EMP 231.31

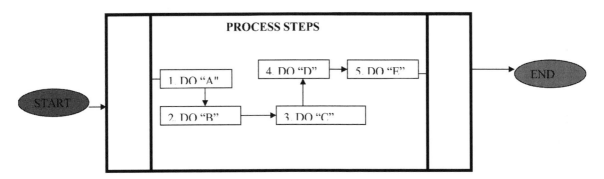

Each process in a second-level map should have a process flow map. A process flow depicts steps through which tasks in an individual process are accomplished. The end result of all task accomplishment is process output—the intended end result for the customer of that process.

Each process in your CAPA subsystem should have departmental work instructions. Your work instructions should be numbered according to your documentation system.

Finally, determine what the quality records (proof that action was taken and results were obtained) per process are. These should end up on a quality record matrix. The matrix should show, among other things:

- The CAPA process
- Document description
- Document number
- Department
- Ownership
- Revision level

■ CHAPTER 12:
DOCUMENT MATRIX

Most CAPA system document hierarchy follows the ISO 9001 model: a common-sense business approach. At the top of the pyramid is the CAPA policy, outlining the road map that the organization follows; the second layer outlines the workflow between departments; the third layer lays out how tasks get accomplished in individual departments; and the last layer comprises CAPA records, or the proof of what was done.

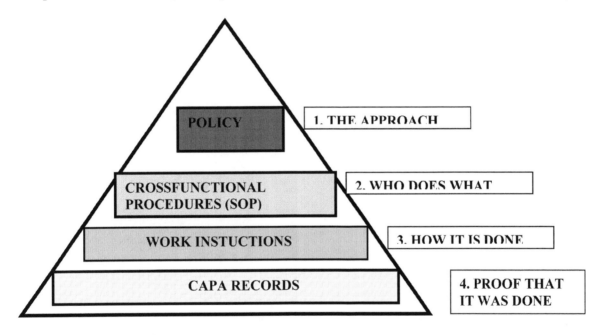

Policies are by nature very high -level documents. They provide a general blueprint, mission, or purpose of the CAPA system. Your policy should be representative of your high-level system map. A policy should never exceed two pages in length.

1. CAPA POLICY: Approach/Roadmap (High-Level Map)

This is the piece that outlines the organization's general approach to solving problems and potential problems through the CAPA system. It is by nature a high-level map that paints the picture in the form of phases through which work gets accomplished. It is a level one document that spells out the roadmap for continuous improvement.

ESSENTIAL ELEMENTS OF A CAPA POLICY DOCUMENT
While slight variations may exist in style and format, the following elements are essential
for any CAPA policy:

- Purpose/mission
- Scope
- Document number
- Document references
- Responsibilities/ownership
- Version control number

SCOPE: Establishes boundaries around affected organizational units. It is very
important to establish boundaries. This stops the ball from dropping between
departments, since CAPA is by default a cross-functional subsystem.

DOCUMENT NUMBER: Establishes traceability and version control.

REFERENCES: Establishes the cross-functional nature of the departments involved;
also document linkages.

RESPONSIBILITIES: Establishes process ownership.

PURPOSE/MISION: Establishes the blueprint /the approach to be followed in
executing the policy.

AN EXAMPLE OF A CAPA POLICY

1.0 TITLE: Amana Biomedical Services' Corrective Action and Preventive Action Policy.
2.0 PURPOSE: To establish a framework through which problems and potential problems
related to the QMS, processes, and product are discovered, investigated, controlled, reviewed,
resolved, and monitored throughout the organization.
3.0 MISSION: It is the policy of Amana Biomedical Services to continuously improve the
Quality Management System through the discovery of problems and potential problems
associated with product, process, and QMS. Containing potential problems and actual
problems, investigating them, reviewing them, and controlling them.

2.0 SCOPE: This policy refers to problems and potential problems identified in the
following quality subsystems:

    2.1 Supplier management
    2.2 Production and process control
    2.3 Change management
    2.4 Facilities
    2.5 Training
    2.6 Management review
    2.7 Design review

2.8 Service records
2.9 Audits
2.10 Design validation
2.11 Quality assurance
2.12 Change control

3.0 RESPONSIBILITIES:

The CAPA system is the responsibility of the quality manager, CAPA administrator, director change management, process engineering manager, manufacturing manager, inventory control manager, material control, customer management and purchasing.

4.0 REFERENCES:

This policy applies to the following documents:
4.1 MPP 003 Auditing the quality system
4.2 STP 001 Policy on supplier audits
4.3 MXC 004 Equipment validation
4.4 MNPS 005 Manufacturing instruction policy
4.5 PRC 002 Process control policy
4.6 QCI 007 Quality control indices
4.7 ECP 009 Equipment calibration
4.8 TRR004 Policy on training; training records
4.9 CC007 Change control policy

5.0 RECORDS

The following documents will store information on actions taken in the execution of this policy:
1.1 Customer complaint record
1.2 Process control charts
1.3 Corrective Action Requests
1.4 Preventive Action Requests
1.5 Investigation reports
1.6 Status reports
1.7 Escalation reports
1.8 Management review reports
1.9 Annual review reports
6.0 Suspension of activities report
7.0 Material review reports
8.0 Closure reports
9.0 Process audit records
10.0 Change control records

DOC.QAP 0947. Rev 001/0504.

2. AN EXAMPLE OF SECOND-LAYER DOCUMENTS: INTER -DEPARTMENT WORK FLOW DOCUMENTS

1.0 Purpose: This document outlines the method through which a Corrective Action Request (CAR) or a Preventive Action request (PAR) is initiated between departments upon the discovery of a problem or potential problem.

2.0 SCOPE: This document applies to the following quality units:
2.1 Auditing
2.2 Process engineering
2.3 Customer management
2.4 Purchasing
2.5 Inventory control
2.6 Manufacturing
2.7 Supplier management
2.8 Quality assurance
2.9 Quality control
2.10 Information management

3.0 REFFERENCE:
The following documents should be referred to in addition to this procedure:
AUD 712 Audit procedures
QA 091 Quality assurance procedures
PR O718 Process engineering processes
QRE 0768 Discovery phase process map

4.0 PROCEDURE:
4.1 Auditor logs the discrepancy on form QAM 0710 per Doc 817.7.
4.2 QC determines if preventive action or corrective action is needed per Doc MPC 078.
4.3 QC completes form QA 11 for Preventive Action Request, and form QA12 for Corrective Action Request, as specified in MMPC 091.
4.4 QC forwards the request to responsible department head per MMP 011.
4.5 Department head forwards CAP or PAP to QC per QA 002.
4.6 QC approves CAP or PAP per QA 00198.
4.7 QC assigns CAR or PAR number and forwards the CAR or PAR to information management system per QA 0070.

DOC.QP0017.Rev 003/0204

3. EXAMPLE OF WORK INSTRUCTIONS: Level three documents

1.0 PROCESS: INITIATION OF A CORRECTIVE ACTION REQUEST

2.0 PURPOSE: Procedure for completing a Corrective Action Request (CAR) or a Preventive Action Request (PAR).

4.0 SCOPE: This procedure applies to all personnel authorized to complete CARs and PARs.

5.0 REFERENCE:
In addition to this work instruction, the following documents should be used as reference:
QA1178 Audit system
PE 908 Process control
PE 1119 Incoming material control

6.0 DEFINITIONS:
6.1 CARs: Corrective Action Requests
6.2 PARs: Preventive Action Requests

7.0 METHOD:
7.1Complete part A of form PCQ1008.
7.2 Define the problem in Part B of the form.
7.3 Attach relevant information.
7.4 Classify the problem/potential problem.
7.5 Assign the correct problem code in Part D.
7.6 Forward the CAR/PAR to the department head responsible.

DOC. QA1174 /0204 Rev.4001

4. AN EXAMPLE OF FOURTH-LAYER DOCUMENT:
Record, proof of action taken and traceability

TITTLE: CAPA PROGRESS REPORT

DATE	CA #	PA #	ISSUE	PROCESS	PRODUCT	QMS	STATUS	OWNER
11/23/2002	1237		Process parameter fluctuation	X			Investigation	PE
12/20/2003		4317	Increased customer returns		X		Escalation	QC
12/24/2003	347		Customer complaint		x		CLOSSED	QC
12/24/2004		5423	Increased Equipment down-time	X			OPEN	Facilities
12/30/2004	376		Increased particle count in clean room	X			Management review	PE AND Facilities
12/30/2004	470 *FDA 483		Ineffective change control subsystem			x	Management Review	VP QUALITY
12/30/2004	472 *FDA 483		Failure to maintain equipment	X			Escalation	VP QUALITY
	QA0452002Re2							

All the documents written for your CAPA system should be numbered according to your numbering system and recorded on your CAPA document matrix.

CAPA MASTER DOCUMENT MATRIX

DOCUMENT NUMBER	DOCUMEENT DESCRIPTION	PROCESS	REVISIONS LEVEL
1.MPO 090	CAPA policy	All	3 6/20/04
2.QP 0017	Departmental instructions	1. CAR initiation	3 02/11/04
3.PE 1170	Departmental instructions	2. Assigning Risk	1 12/20/04
4.QA 1122	Departmental instructions	3. Investigation	1 11/11/03
5.IT 1567	Work instructions	Logging	1
6.PE 111	Work instructions	Team formation	1
8.QA 1174	Work instructions	1. CAR initiation	1
9. PE 090	Work instructions	Investigation	1
10.QA 002	Departmental workflow	Investigation	1
11. QA0007	Record	CA approval	1
12. QA 04520	Record	Status Report	1

CHAPTER: 13:
CAPA VOCABULARY

Like any system, the CAPA system has its own language, and a list of all the terms used should be made available to the users of the system. Though ISO 1804 could be used as a reference for your definitions, the responsibility of developing the CAPA lexicon is left entirely to the organization. My advice to all my customers is always "Just make sure you are speaking the same language as the FDA." Their definitions are in harmony with ISO definitions. Here is a partial list of some of the definitions of words and acronyms you might need. They are not carved in stone.

A

1. **Analysis:** Documentation demonstrating that data were analyzed for possible unfavorable trends or other indicators of product, process, or quality system.
2. **Audit:** A systematic, independent, and documented process of obtaining evidence and evaluating it objectively to determine the extent to which criteria are fulfilled.
3. **Audit** findings: Results of the evaluation of the collected audit evidence against audit criteria.
4. **Assignable cause**: Source of variation that is intermittent and unpredictable.

B

1. **Bimodial Distribution**: A distribution curve with two identifiable curves within it, indicating the presence of two assignable causes.

C.

1. **CFR:** An acronym for Code Of Federal Requirements.
2. **Correction:** A one-time action taken to eliminate a detected non-conformity. It is usually a temporary solution to an event. Re-work is perceived as correction of a problem.
3. **CAPA:** An acronym for Corrective Action and Preventive Action.
4. **Corrective Action**: An action taken to eliminate causes of an actual problem. The action is aimed at preventing recurrence of the problem.
5. **Compliance:** Affirmation that the supplier of a product or service has made requirements of the relevant specifications or regulations.

6. **Concession:** Permission to use or release a product that does not conform to specified requirements, e.g. "use as is."
7. **Control Chart**: A graphic representation of a characteristic of a process, showing plotted values of some statistic gathered from that characteristic, as well as control limits.
8. **Cost of Quality**: "Total cost of doing things wrong." It includes the cost of re-work, scrap, rejects, customer returns, and equipment downtime.
9. **CAR:** An acronym for Corrective Action Request.
10. **Conformance** : An affirmative indication or judgment that a product or service has met the requirements of the relevant specifications or regulations. It also means the state of meeting requirements.
11. **Control limit**: Lines on a control chart used to judge the significance of variation.
12. **CAP:** Corrective action plan.

D.

1. **Deviation:** Not following set instructions or set standard operating procedures.
2. **Planned Deviation**: A planned exception to the standard way of doing things. Requesting for a variance in process parameters so product can be re-worked is a planned deviation. A Deviation Request to deviate from standard operating procedures for a particular lot is an example of a planned deviation.
3. **Unplanned** Deviation: Operating contrary to the organization's standard operating procedures.
4. **Discrepancy:** Not meeting set standards.
5. **Design validation**: Test to insure that the product conforms to defined user needs.
6. **Design of experiments (DOE)**: Manipulating controllable factors to see their effects on process outputs.
7. **Defect:** The non-fulfillment of intended usage requirements.
8. **Design Review**: A formal, documented, comprehensive, and systematic examination of a design to evaluate design requirements and capability.

E.

1. **Escalation:** Elevation of an issue to a higher decision-making level for review due to recurrence, failure to take action, or failure of effective check.
2. **Effectiveness check**: A documented process that establishes that an action taken was effective and accomplished the objective it was intended for.
3. **Event:** Any discrepancy that may affect product or process and requires correction to be controlled. Discovery of non-conforming products among shipped on a customer cite (an event) may lead to a recall of several lots of the product (correction).
4. **ECN:** An acronym for Engineering Change Notice.
5. **ECO:** An acronym for Engineering Change Order.

F

1. **FMEA:** Failure mode and effects analysis. A method for determining the level of risk involved. Two types exist: PFMEA (Process FMEA) and DFMEA (Design FMEA).
2. **FTA:** Fault tree analysis.

G.

cGMP: Current Good Manufacturing Practices. Federal guidelines for FDA regulated industries.

L.

LOOP: Naturally occurring cycles in any system which counter the effects of each other to restore equilibrium in that system. In a CAPA system, the preventive loop counters the effects of the corrective loop to restore equilibrium in the cost of quality.

M

1. **Management Review**: A systematic activity that the executive management of an organization carries out to evaluate the adequacy and status of the QMS.
2. **Management representative with authority**: A member of the management team who is responsible for decision making.
3. **Material Review Board (MRB)**: A quality board that works on material dispositions.

N

1. **Non-conformance:** Failing to meet requirements or set specifications.
2. **Non-conforming material**: Any raw material that fails to meet set specifications.
3. **Non-conforming product**: Any products that do not meet customer requirements.
4. **Non-conformity:** The non-fulfillment of a requirement.

O

1. **Output:** The end product of a process.
2. **Out of specification**: Not meeting specifications.
3. **OCAP:** An acronym for Out-of-Control Action Plan.

P

1. **Preventive Action**: An action taken to eliminate the cause of potential non-conformity. The action is taken to stop occurrence of the potential problem.
2. **Process:** A set of interrelated steps that add value on an input to produce a desired output.

3. **Process parameters**: Set conditions at which the process operates. They are the upper control limit (UCL), low control limit (LCL), and the Control Limit (CL).
4. **Parts per million (PPM)**: A way used to state the performance of a process in terms of actual defective products.
5. **Process capability**: The measure in reproducibility of the product turned out by the process using normal distribution.
6. **Process validation**: Establishing by objective evidence that a process consistently produces a result or product meeting predetermined specifications.
7. **PAR:** An acronym for Preventive Action Request.
8. **Process map**: Sequence of events in a process that add value to an input to produce an output.

Q

1. **QMS:** Acronym for the Quality Management System.
2. **Quality:** The characteristics of an entity that address the ability of that entity to satisfy given needs.
3. **Quality management system (QMS)**: Organizational structures, procedures, processes, and resources needed to accomplish the overall intention of the organization.
4. **Quality control unit**: An operational unit responsible for activities that monitor processes for unsatisfactory performance and continuous improvement.
5. **Quality Assurance**: Planned activities within the QMS which provide confidence that the product will fulfill the customer's requirements. An example here would be final inspection.
6. **Quality system review**: Annual review of quality system indicators.
7. **Quality Audit**: A systematic, independent evaluation to determine whether quality activities and related results comply with written requirements and whether the requirements achieve stated objectives.
8. **QSR:** Quality system regulations.

R

1. **Root-cause analysis**: A systematic method used to get to the assignable cause of system, product, or processes non-conformity. It examines the effects of man, method, machine, material, and Mother Nature, or environment, on the final effect.
2. **Root cause**: The underlying factor or assignable cause of the problem.
3. **Record:** Documentation that provides both the results achieved in an activity and the evidence that the activity took place.
4. **Requirement:** Stated needs or expectations.

S

1. **Satellite system**: A quality management subsystem that feeds quality information into the CAPA system through discovery vehicles.

2. **Second-level map**: Sequential workflows between departments in an organization that establishes ownership.

3. **System:** A set of interrelated processes that act together as a whole to produce a desired result over time.

4. **System loop**: Natural and dynamic cycles in any system, which counterbalance the effects of each other to restore equilibrium. Spending time and money by proactively catching problems before they occur lowers the time and money the organization spends reacting to problems when they occur.

5. **Supplier:** The provider of an input for a process, or an internal customer in a system.

T.

1. **Trend:** A sequence or pattern of data. Trend analysis helps detect the root cause of a problem.

V

1. **Variance:** A planned deviation or non-conformance that may be requested for special cases like re-work. Variances are a one-time event. They should be tracked through the CAPA system.

2. **Validation:** Confirming that requirements have been made through the examination of objective evidence.

3. **Verification:** Auditing per requirements for confirmation.

■ CHAPTER 14:
INFORMATION
MANAGEMENT SYSTEM

The next step should be finding an information management system to support your designed system. There are several companies out there that have products on the market that are claimed to be 21 CFR Part 11 compliant. Those products range from window-based tracking software to full-fledged web-enabled systems. When it comes to information management systems, no one system fits all organizations. Choose a system that is 21CFR Part 11 compliant, meets the needs of your organization, and is configurable enough to support your process flows and the existing infrastructure. The following is a list of information system requirements that were introduced to you in chapter six. Whatever your information system requirements may be, incorporate 21 CFR Part 11 in your requirements as the bare minimum requirements that your system must meet.

INFORMATION MANAGEMENT SYSTEM REQUIMENTS

It is imperative to have an information management system for your CAPA system, not only for traceability and accountability purposes, but also to have customer and supplier involvement in problem solving and quality improvement in your organization. The idea is to have collaboration in quality improvement between suppliers of materials to your organization, end users of your products, and your organization itself. For that reason, it is recommended that your information management system meet the following conditions:

(a) Be web-based. In this kind of system, all that is needed is a web browser. Most computers are sold with this "gizmo" anyway. No extra expense here.
(b) Not be client/server technology requiring application-specific software that requires configuration on client computers.
(c) Be able to provide real-time information and analyses, to cut down on response time on critical situations like recalls, quarantine, and containment.
(d) Be part of your core information system, not a QA database.
(e) Work across all types of operating systems and platforms, including Windows, Mac, UNIX, Linux, Solaris and Palm.
(f) Offre easy configuration and customization of forms, fields, workflows and security settings.
(g) Be easily integrated with other information systems already installed in your organization.

(h) Have bulletproof security with limited access to users and departments, such as thwarting repeated attempts to gain unauthorized access, and immediate notification to the system administrator of the threat.

(I) Allow for file attachments and storage.

(j) Have a universal email integration capability.

(k) Allow for definitions for task escalation to management.

(l) Be 21 CFR Part 11 compliant. This requirement governs electronic records and electronic signatures. In summary, to be Part 11 compliant, your system should have the following capabilities:

- A secure time-stamped audit trail of all actions taken
- Application of signatures only by genuine owners
- Password protection
- Session time-out
- Lock-out upon failed login attempts
- Activity history of all actions taken
- Different authorization levels

(m) Have graphical statistical analysis capability.

(n) Have reports and graph generation capability.

CHAPTER 15:
VALIDATION

A dry run of all your CAPA processes should be performed once all your processes are in place and your information system is up and running. There are several process validation protocols out there. The aim of process validation is to insure that the design meets set objectives. In other words, you should make sure that all processes are working the way they were set up to operate. Where a discrepancy from the expected results presents itself, an engineering change order should be requested. Below is a recommended path to follow:

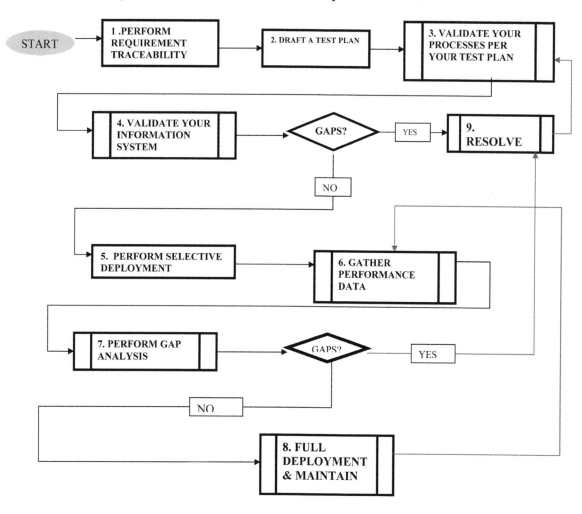

1. PERFORMING REQUIREMENT TRACEABILITY

Audit all your pour system against the requirements you set up. At a minimum, your processes and information management system should meet all regulatory requirements. You should be able to pinpoint where in your system a particular requirement is met.

2. DRAFTING A TEST PLAN

In drafting a test plan for your system, the focus should be on the mission of your CAPA system: what the system is supposed to achieve for the organization and how it is supposed to achieve that end. The second part should be focused on system suppliers, inputs, and customer requirements.

3. PROCESS VALIDATION

It is imperative to make sure that all processes in your system meet their objectives, and that there are no gaps (the ball is not being dropped anywhere) in your system. There are many models for process validation. Pick one that works for you.

4. VALIDATION OF THE INFORMATION MANAGEMENT SYSTEM

The key here is validation of your software and hardware. The second item that should be of concern to you should be Part 11 compliance.

5. SELECTIVE DEPLOYMENT

It is recommended that before full rollout a partial deployment be done. For multi-site organizations, it is recommended that selective deployment be done on one site to test the culture and infrastructure of your organization. For smaller organizations, selective deployment may be limited to trained personnel only.

6. DATA GATHERING:

Develop system performance matrix. You have to come up with the measure for your system performance. The first step is to determine what to measure, how to measure it, and when to measure it. The second step is to analyze that data and establish your baseline.

7. FILL THE GAPS

Fine-tune your system to run the way it is supposed to run by addressing issues that have been discovered before proceeding to full deployment.

8. FULL DEPLOYMENT

Full deployment should only take place when all personnel have been trained to use the system. It is important that system performance data is kept to feed the continuous improvement loop.

Once a partial deployment has been made, draft a responsibility matrix for all processes and all the personnel involved in the operation of your CAPA system. Launch a full-scale training program for all the parties on your matrix, and make roles and responsibilities very clear in your responsibility matrix.

RESPONSIBILITY MATRIX

PROCESS	OWNERSHIP	RESPONSIBILITY
1. QUALITY RECORD REVIEW	1. INTERNAL AUDITOR 1. EXTERNAL AUDITOR	1. AUDIT FINDING REVIEW 1. AUDIT REVIEW
2. CAR/PAR APPROVAL	2. QA MANAGER	2. APPROVE CAR/PAR
3. PRIORITY ASSIGNMENT	3. CAPA ADMIN	3. ASSIGN PRIORITY AND OWNERSHIP
4. RISK ANALYSIS	4. QUALITY AND PROCESS ENGINEERING	4. ASSESS RISK
5. NON-CONFORMING PRODUCT CONTROL	5. INVENTORY CONTROL/ MRB	5. GAIN CONTROL OF NON-CONFORMING PRODUCTS
6. RISK CONTAINMENT	6. QUALITY ENGINEERING	6. CORRECTION OF EVENTS
7. ROOT CAUSE ANALYSIS	7. QUALITY COUNCIL	7. INVESTIGATION
8. IMPLEMENTATION OF BEST SOLUTIONS	8. QUALITY COUNCIL	8. IMPLEMENTATION
9. VALIDATION OF BEST SOLUTIONS	9. QUALITY CONTROL AND PROCESS CONTROL	9. VALIDATE BEST SOLUTION PRIOR TO IMPLEMENTATION
10. CAPA CLOSURE	10. QUALITY CONTROL	10. DRAFT CLOSURE REPORT
11. ESCALATION RECORD REVIEW	11. VP QUALITY	11. MANAGEMENT REVIEW, DISPOSITION, AND RESOURCE ALLOCATION.

CHAPTER 16:
SYSTEM METRICS

The final step in your design is to come up with health indicators for your system. CAPA indicators tell you whether your system is accomplishing what it was designed to accomplish or not. To choose good health indicators, you must revisit the mission of a CAPA system in chapter one.

CAPA MISSION SUMMARY

Here is what a CAPA system is supposed to accomplish:

Subpart J 820.00(a) (1) summary: The system should be able to do the following:

Perform analysis of processes, work operations, concessions, audit records, service records, customer complaints, returned products, and other quality data to identify existing and potential causes of non-conforming products and other quality problems, using statistical methodology.

In other words, if your CAPA system accomplishes the above mission, your organization should not:

1. Spend most of its resources reacting to events
2. Have high concession numbers
3. Have high cost of scrap
4. Have high cost of re-work
5. Have high equipment downtime due to corrective maintenance
6. Have high customer returns
7. Have legal penalties
8. Have high cost of warranties
9. Have high reject rates at final inspection due to inherent variation
10. Have decreased market share
11. Have low customer retention ratio due to dissatisfaction
12. Have increased cycle time due to process down time
13. Have regulatory and external audit findings
14. Have dissatisfied customers

The list of indices you can monitor is based on the outputs of the conformance triangle: process, product, and quality management system. A stable and predictable process produces products that are consistent in quality and requirements. A customer whose needs and requirements are met by an organization does not have anything to complain about—hence, low customer returns, high rate in customer retention, and an increased market share. These are indices of the effectiveness of your overall quality management system. Your CAPA matrix should be representative of these indices.

An example of a CAPA matrix is given below:

CAPA MATRIX

What do we measure to know how good our system is at finding problems and potential problems and solving them to restore equilibrium in our quality management system? This should be your question while determining your matrix. Here is an example of indices you should look at as a measure of efficiency:

MONTH	CAPA INDICATOR.						
	1. COST OF EVENTS $	2. IN-PROCESS REJECTS $	3. CUSTOMER RETURNS $	4. AVERAGE CUSTOMER RETENTION (YRS.)	5. EQUIPMENT DOWN TIME (HOURS)	6. REJECTS AT FINAL $	7. EXTERNAL AUDIT FINDINGS FDA 483s,and Warning letters QTY.
JANUARY							
FEBRUARY							
MARCH							
APRIL							
MAY							
JUNE							
JULY							
AUGUST							
SEPTEMBER							
OCTOBER							
NOVEMBER							
DECEMBER							
QUARTERLY AVERAGE							
ANNUAL AVERAGE							

As a rule of thumb, pick at a minimum six indicators: Two process-related, two product-related, and two quality system management-related. The indices "reject at final" and "customer returns" are considered product-related. Since the cost of events and customer retention are cumulative in nature, they are considered QMS-related. Equipment downtime and in-process rejects are considered process-related. The emphasis, again, is on the preventive loop. If you catch potential problems before they turn into problems, you won't spend resources reacting to problems. In essence, prevention cost less than cure. That is why we have HMOs (Health Maintenance Organizations) and car maintenance programs! The same applies to a quality management system. Prevention is always better than cure!

REFERENCE:

1. *Code of federal regulations, 21CFR parts 200 to 1299.*
   National Archives and Records Administration.
   Washington D.C: GPO, April 1,20002.

2. Parch, Robert. *The ISO 900 Handbook*
   New York: McGraw-Hill, 2000.

3. Nevalainen, David, Lucia Berte and Marjana F.Callery.
   Quality Systems in the Blood Bank Environment. Bethesda, Maryland: American
   Association of Blood Banks, 1998.

TAKE THE INITIATIVE!

Here is a little story about four people named Everybody, Anybody, Somebody, and Nobody. There was an important job to be done, and Everybody thought Somebody would do it. As it turned out, Nobody did it, and Somebody got ticked off because it was Everybody's job, and Anybody could have done it!

Quality is everybody's job!

Modified from, Author unknown.

NOTES

NOTES

NOTES

NOTES

NOTES

6954135R0

Made in the USA
Lexington, KY
06 October 2010